May Magee

GW00420142

STEP BY STEP
AROMATHERAPY

A simple step by step, easy to follow, guide which explains the principles and applications of Aromatherapy

Douglas Barry Publications
21 Laud Street
Croydon
Surrey
CR0 1SU

AROMATHERAPY MASSAGE
A HANDBOOK FOR EVERYONE

FIRST PUBLISHED IN THE U.K. 1992

STEP BY STEP
AROMATHERAPY

Reprint 1992
Reprint 1993

British Library - A CIP Catalogue
record for this book is available
from the British Library.

I.S.B.N.   0-9516203-2-0
Published in Great Britain by
Douglas Barry Publications,
21 Laud Street,
Croydon, Surrey.
CRO 1SU

DEDICATED TO THE MEMORY OF
MY LATE PARENTS

ACKNOWLEDGEMENTS

I am indebted to many people who assisted me in the writing of this book. Firstly, I would like to thank my family for all the time, energy and constant encouragement given during the writing of the manuscript.

Also my clients, friends and students, both past and present who encouraged me to put my ideas down on paper and without whom this book might never have been written.

To my niece Brenda who despite many operations and the resultant long stays in hospital, has always proved to be nothing short of an inspiration to me.

I wish to place on record my thanks and appreciation for the help, support and encouragement given to me by my friend Anneke Van der Mey.

My thanks also to Eleanor Gash and Jane Bond for their advice and comment.

Finally, the input of R and S cannot be ignored.

CONTENTS

FORWARD

My own Beauty Therapy and Aromatherapy teacher, the late Marion Ayers, was a lady ahead of her time. Her school being one of, if not the first in the U.K. She predicted in the early sixties the Common Market and all the changes which have now taken place in the field of Beauty and Complementary Medicine.

Her childhood was a sickly one. She spent a lot of her formative years confined to bed; which was probably a contributory factor to her great understanding of people, their way of thinking and how the mind and surroundings can have a great influence on our general state of health and wellbeing. Marion's forward thinking earned her the title, in those days, of being an eccentric. If only those who gave her that title could have been blessed with her foresight and abilities perhaps Complementary Therapies would have been on today's professional footing a long time ago.

She was a great admirer and student of the work of Renée Gattefosse. She also exchanged ideas with Marguerite Maury who she invited me to meet when I attended seminars on Aromatherapy and 'The Prescription Mix', as she would call the individual blending recipes. My own interest in the oils grew almost daily but I felt starved of information, although I read every book on herbs, plants and ancient remedies that I could find. Literally it was often a case of searching through old bric-a-brac shops and library cast outs.

Marion encouraged me to go to Paris where I was given the

1

opportunity to work for a short time as a beauty therapist and to improve my skills as a massage therapist. The product used for massage was essential oil based, pre-prepared in the laboratory. We were encouraged to study the history and chemical composition of plants and oils, as was customary practice for therapists with all product ingredients.

I returned to Marion in the mid sixties for a further period of training in the use of essential oils which included training in the preparation of creams, lotions and ointments, using essential oils which she had obtained from Marguerite Maury. Again Marion asked me to go to Europe for experience; this time I travelled to Italy and Portugal. As an Irish country girl I already had the experience of growing up with and loving the wonders of nature. The late sixties and early seventies took me to Holland where I worked as an aromatherapist (mainly for Americans and overseas groups in the chemical industry). After which, on a trip to Africa, I continued the use of essential oils and Beauty Therapy while adding Reflexology to my skills.

My love for Aromatherapy and standards for training have not waned through the years. I have taken advantage of every opportunity to advance my knowledge, which, in itself, says something for that now almost forgotten English lady who gave so much to so many, Marion Ayers. If she was alive today she would be unable to read this tribute to her greatness as she was blind for a number of years prior to her death in the early eighties.

In the seventies I opened my Beauty Therapy Training School which also offers courses in Massage, Aromatherapy and Reflexology. This is when this book began its life in the form of notelets/handouts. The urgency to complete my task of putting the notelets into print (this book) was soon relieved by a very young and then almost unheard of author, Robert Tisserand. My notes became the students' bible and Robert's book The Art of Aromatherapy, their prayers. Through constant study and now research Aromatherapy has become a household name. My hope is that teachers and therapists will be responsible people and that the public will be made aware of the dangers, as well as the benefits, of Essential Oils. Like most professions our own has not been spared the charlatan training centres and therapists, who have neither the knowledge nor experience to work with members of the public and, worse still, charge fees for so doing. The day is drawing very near when all therapists working with members of the public will be accountable to a professional body for their actions; a situation long awaited by the many good training centres and professional therapists.

Renée Tanner

WHAT IS AROMATHERAPY?

When we speak of aromatherapy we are not just talking about massage but of the various methods and uses of **essential oils for the good of the recipient.**

Aroma meaning 'sweet smelling' and therapy meaning 'with intent to heal'.

It is important before using essential oils that the properties are known, as some of the oils can be harmful to use in certain conditions; some can even be skin irritants. Just because they are natural doesn't mean they are all harmless.

The oils are obtained from flowers, leaves, plants and trees.

The powerful therapeutic healing properties of the oils are used in many ways but principally in massage, compress, inhalation and baths.

WHAT ARE ESSENTIAL OILS?

The aromatherapist uses essential oils blended in a base or carrier (blending varies depending on age, condition or illness). The essential oil is a complex substance extracted from a plant. This substance contains the greatest part of the therapeutic properties of a plant though not necessarily all of them.

Plants have naturally occurring substances which we call essences (they are often thought of as being the life force of the plant). When these essences are submitted to certain processes an essential oil is produced. In other words, essential oils are not naturally occurring in plants in the form used by the therapist, but become essential oils when the essences are extracted from the plant by means of **distillation**. Because of this process the essential oil is not identical to the essence.

The compounds which go to make up the plant essence are produced in special cells called secretory cells. These cells are usually near the surface and are grouped together to form the secretory glands which store the oil/essence; however this does depend to some extent on the type of plant, as some plants have a secretory sac or duct for storage. These secretory cells can be found in virtually any part of the plant e.g. leaves, flowers, bark, fruits, roots, stem or seeds. Some plants even produce different essences in different parts of the same plant; one such example being the orange tree.
From the petals we get neroli.
From the leaves we get petitgrain.
From the orange fruit rind we get orange.

It is important for all users of essential oil to know the part of the plant used to obtain the oil as there may be differences in the therapeutic effect of oils from different parts of the same plant (for example the oil from the Juniper berry is superior to that of the leaves of the plant). For safety sake it is also worth bearing in mind that to use the full botanical - Latin name of the required oil is quite important in order to avoid any misunderstandings. It is also worthwhile confirming with the supplier that the oils are pure, unadulterated and unstretched. This is especially important for the professional aromatherapist if buying oils outside the normal sphere of the profession.

Professional aromatherapists will usually not be in the position of having to buy oils over the counter where perhaps temperature and storage might not be ideal.

A HISTORY OF AROMATHERAPY THROUGH THE AGES

The first step in the history of Aromatherapy is probably almost as old as man himself. It is impossible to date when flowers, plants and roots were first used for medicinal purposes.

Early man discovered that some of the branches and twigs that he burnt on his fire for warmth caused changes in mood; some giving feelings of wellbeing, some giving feelings of drowsiness. Inevitably they realised that the aromas of the smoke helped with difficult breathing and congestion.

Early man depended on Nature's larder of fruits, berries, roots and leaves not only for the food he ate but to cure the sick and heal his wounds. It is also feasible that he gained some of his knowledge of the benefits of plants by studying sick animals to see what they ate and how they reacted. As the reason behind the healing properties of plants was unknown, the communities tended to attribute the process to a God or Gods. Styrax was linked with Saturn, Costus with Mars, Myrrh with the Moon, and Incense with the Sun. Osiers was the God of Vegetation and his twin sister had the power to renew life.

THE EGYPTIANS

To the ancient Egyptians medicine was a way of life. They are known to have used Myrrh, Frankincense, Cedarwood, Origanum, Bitter Almond, Spikenard, Henna, Juniper, Coriander and Calamus. Their love of flowers is depicted in many of their earliest wall paintings.

Various medical papyri dating back to 2000 B.C. were discovered by archeologists in the last 100 years and these list a number of recipes in use after 1800 B.C. the majority being of vegetable base. Each recipe described the condition as well as its symptoms and gave clear instructions on how the medication should be prepared and administered.

Plants and herbs were used not only for medicinal purposes but were also for embalming the dead. This showed great knowledge of plants and herbs as well as of anatomy.

Cedarwood was one of the oils used in mummification. Its use can be attributed to the fact that it was considered to be imperishable. Several centuries later the mummified bodies found in the tombs were well preserved and this has been attributed to the antibacterial and antiseptic properties of the oils.

The Egyptians used infused oils. They also used a form of Enfleurage to extract their oils. It is quite possible to assume from some of the findings and records, that the Egyptians practised a method of distillation. Should this prove to be true distillation would have been known to the Egyptians at least 2000 years before the Arabians were supposed to have invented the process.

The Egyptians treated hayfever with a mixture of antimony, aloes, myrrh and honey and went on to discover a spermicide which was a blend of acacia coloquinte, dates and honey.

Kyphi or Khypi, the oldest form of perfume known to man, (a mixture of sixteen different oils) was very popular with the Egyptians both in the home and for use by the priests in the temples. When archeologists opened the tomb of Tutankhamun (reign 1361-1352 B.C.) in 1922 the smell of Kyphi was said to have emanated from it. The archeologists found scent pots and vases, some contained ungents (an ointment). Although the scent was faint it was still detectable, later it was possible to establish the identity of some of the contents of the pots. The tomb had been sealed in 1350 B.C., during the reign of Khufa who built the great Pyramid.

Earlier still when the tomb of King Menes (3000 B.C.) was opened in 1897 it was found to have the remains of aromatic products present.

In 1978 archeologists divulged the secrets of Queen Nefertiti's beauty. It is said that she used beauty cleansing masks of honey, milk and flower pollens. To keep her skin soft, she also bathed in a bath containing oils from eighty different fruits and herbs as well as using a lotion of honey and orchard leaves. The last Queen of Egypt, Cleopatra, is said to have seduced Mark Antony by her lavish use of perfume.

MESOPOTAMIA

Mesopotamia (modern Iraq) has a history going back to the Summarians and the Babylonians. The region is one of the earliest centres of civilised life.

The Babylonian doctors recorded their prescriptions on clay tablets and gave clear details as to when and how a remedy should be prepared and taken. What they did not record, however, was the quantities to be used.

Like the Egyptians the Summarians believed that sickness was the manifestation of devils and evil spirits. What we do not know is who influenced whom in this belief.

Kings of the day established gardens of medicinal plants. Many of these plants are still in use today; they include : Apricot, Myrrh, Poppy, Sesame, Garlic, Onion, Fennel, Rose, Juniper.

ANCIENT GREECE

This ancient civilization took much from the Egyptian and Mesopotamian worlds including their knowledge of medicine. This gave the Greeks great stepping stones for advancement in making further discoveries as well as laying the foundations for a scientific basis to medicine.

They used perfumed oils for cosmetic and medicinal purposes. Soldiers were given ointment of Myrrh to carry with them to help heal the wounds of war.

Marestheus, a Greek physician, recognised that aromatic plants and flowers had either stimulating or sedative properties.

Theophrastus, - Father of Botany, recommended the use of olive oil to absorb the perfume of the aromatic oil as this prolonged the life of the scent.

Hippocrates, - Father of medicine (460 - 377 BC) was the first person known to establish and set down a scientific system of medicine, a system of diagnosis and prognosis. He used over 400 drugs of vegetable origin in his prescriptions and studies.

Excerpts from Hippocritical collection :

Hippocrates made a statement claiming that "there is a cure in earth for every ill".

"A wise man ought to realise that health is his most valuable possession and learn how to treat illnesses by his own judgement".

Many famous Greeks worked for the Romans.
Galen,- Born 13 AD in Turkey (which was then under Greek rule), he was physician to Marcus Aurelius and was the first physician to diagnose the pulse; he is also credited with the original Cold Cream. An outstanding writer, Galen recorded a great deal on the theory of plant medicine and plant classification.

Dioscorides - The chief physician to Nero, had by 78 AD collected information on plants all around the Mediterranean.

He left us his recordings in "Materia Medica" which contained information not only on the plants but also their uses. He praised the onion for its diuretic and tonic properties and its effectiveness against infection.

Centuries later his theories about the onion were proved in that its juices worked as an antibiotic against staphylococcus and other microbes. Onion has also been used by the Australian aborigines to ward off infection.

Pliny - His encyclopedia of 37 volumes had no less than 16 volumes devoted to plants. His works represented the writings and findings of almost 400 different authors and although they contained much misinformation they also contained a lot of information that would otherwise have been unavailable to us, as many of the previous studies to which he referred have been destroyed.

The fall of the Roman Empire around 400 AD caused Roman physicians to flee to Constantinople; from here their knowledge was passed to the Arabs.

THE ARABIANS

Although it is customary to speak of Arabian medicine in this period, not all physicians of the day were Arabs or natives. Neither were they all Muslims, some were Jews and some Christians. They were drawn from all areas of the empire stretching along the entire coast of Africa and into Spain. As the great traders they spread their knowledge through the world of the day. The Arabs discovered alcohol, which meant that perfumes could be made without a heavy oil base.

Aly-Ali-Ibn-Sina, more commonly known as Avicenna (980-1037 AD), - is considered to have been one of the greatest Arab physicians. Some say that if Hippocrates is thought of as the father of medicine then surely Avicenna could be considered, amongst other things, to be the Father of Massage and Manipulation. He laid down clear guidelines for massage and originated various forms of manipulations for spinal problems as well as inventing the idea of traction for broken limbs. He was an outstanding scholar, being an accepted doctor by the age of eighteen years. At 21 he was famed for his mastery of formal learning and medical prowess.

He built on the works of Hippocrates, Galen and Dioscorides whose recordings were translated into Persian and other Arab languages. In his own works Avicenna described eight hundred plants and their uses.

In spite of his many achievements, including being made Physician in Chief to a hospital in Bagdad, he was to spend long periods in prison, brought about by the jealousy and intrigue of others. Avicennas's two most famed works were the Book of Healing and Canon of Medicine. He is also credited with having perfected distillation.

EUROPEANS IN GENERAL AND THE MIDDLE AGES

ELEVENTH CENTURY

No real recordings exist between the Eleventh and Twelfth Century; a period known as The Dark Ages.

TWELFTH CENTURY

Knights in the Crusades brought back knowledge of perfumes and how to distil oils. The perfumers of Arabia were now famous throughout Europe. Recipes were available and due to the advent of printing, books called Herbals were printed, giving information on plants and prescriptions.

THIRTEENTH CENTURY

Anaesthetic

The development of distillation was now being encouraged by the new pharmaceutical industry. Not having the same plants as the Orientals the Europeans adapted quickly, using native shrubs and plants; Rosemary, Lavender and Thyme being amongst the many.

The distillation coincided with the achievements of the famous Bologna School of Medicine, which, incidentally, is credited with having contributed greatly to anaesthesia. Their prescription for anaesthetic was to soak into a sponge the juices

14

of plants which had been previously boiled and stored for use.
It is now generally accepted that this method of anaesthetic
originated in India many years before.   During this period St.
Hildegarde, the Abbess of Bingen, wrote four theses on
medicinal plants.   Her works are still referred to today.

THE RENAISSANCE

FOURTEENTH CENTURY   *14 century (Black death)*

In the fourteenth century (1340-1350) the first plague hit
Europe.   Known as The Black Death, it killed almost half of
Europe's population.   The only protection available against
disease, at that time, was the use of aromatic plant material, e.g.
herbs, plants and flowers.   These were strewn onto the floors,
burned in the streets and carried on the person in public in the
form of pomanders.

FIFTEENTH CENTURY

Gildemeister's writings informs us that the oils of Bitter
Almond, Cedar, Cinnamon, Frankincense, Mastic, Rose and
Sage were well known.   During the next two years sixty more
essential oils were added to the list.   J.M. Feminis created the
first Eau Admirable which was further developed by his
nephew and is known today as Eau de Cologne (a proven
antiseptic).

The practice of covering the floor with aromatic plants continued, as did the use of pomanders and lavender bags to ward off disease. In 1492 Columbus landed in the Bahamas. From then on the explorers brought back many herbs, spices and plants.

SIXTEENTH AND SEVENTEENTH CENTURIES

Throughout the middle ages and Tudor times all forms of plant medicine were used by apothecaries, doctors and lay people. This period saw the flourishing growth of the perfumery industry and the periods are noted as the great herbal times of Europe.

The now well established and practiced art of herb-strewing on the floors continued to be enacted to create pleasant smells and help to prevent the spread of disease. The gentlemen of the day, including the medical practitioners, carried a little cassolette filled with aromatics on the top of their walking sticks. This was raised to the nose in the presence of disease or foul smells; it was considered a personal antiseptic. The 17th century has been referred to as the 'Golden age of Herbalists' such as Nicholas Culpeper, John Parkinson, John Gerard in England; Otto Brunfels, Leonard Fuchs and Hieronymus Boch in Germany; Nicholas Monasdes in Spain; Pietro Mattioli in Italy and Charles de l'Ecluse in France.

Culpeper (born 1666) tried to make medicine available to all people and gave treatment free to the poor. He published the English Physician (now known as Culpeper's Herbal) in 1653; it contained 369 medicines made of English herbs. It is believed that Culpeper gained a lot of his knowledge from the writings of Galen.

Mattioli's herbal was translated into a number of European languages and sold 32,000 copies . His work was based on the writings of Dioscorides.

Essential oils were being used not only by herbalists but also by doctors; a trend which continued until the end of the 19th century.

From 1665 to the Great Fire in 1666 there raged the second outbreak of plague. The disease was dealt with in a similar way to that of three hundred years before; it had been noted that the perfumers and those wearing perfumed gloves remained almost immune to the diseases of the time.

One outcome from this tragic time was a growing new science of experimental chemistry; the forerunner to the use of chemical substances in medicine.

THE FAR EAST, INDIA AND CHINA

The use of plants for healing has an unbroken record for thousands of years, unlike Europe, where we are now only beginning to re-discover our broken heritage of knowledge.

17

INDIA

In India the oldest form of medicine is Ayurvedic. Ayur
meaning Life and Veda meaning Knowledge. No synthetic
material is used in this medicine. Ayurvedic is mainly plant
based, although some animal and mineral material is used. In
Ayurveda it is believed that our direct link to the universe
which surrounds us, is through our senses. To feel, to hear, to
see, to smell and taste is to perceive. In India the Lotus
flower grows in abundance along the lakes in Kashmir, where
the flower is the symbol of rejuvenation.

Lord Shiva, one of the Gods of the Hindu faith is referred to
as "The First Herbalist".

Asoka, emperor of India in the 3rd century BC, is said to have
established eighteen institutions, with some characteristics
similar to those of modern hospitals, in that cleanliness was
stressed, diet therapy, as well as treatment with herbs, plants
and oils was practised; but above all patients were treated with
kindness.

He organised and regulated the cultivation of medicinal plants.
Great attention was paid to the conditions in which the plants
grew and to those who tended them. The medicinal plants of
India form the basis of present day traditional medicine in
that country.

CHINA

Like India, China has an unbroken tradition of herbal medicine. The earliest known records are in the "Yellow Emperors' Classics of Internal Medicine" dating back to 2000 BC. It deals mainly with causes and treatment of disease. Another great classic of Chinese herbal medicine known as Pen-Tsao-Khang-Mou, lists 816 different formulae taken from almost 20,000 different substances, most being of plant origin.

The Chinese used opium as a treatment for dysentery from as early as 1000 BC but did not begin to smoke opium until the Ming Dynasty in the sixteenth century when alcohol was banned.

THE 18TH AND 19TH CENTURIES   *synthetic Med*

During the 18th and 19th centuries chemists continued to research the active ingredients of medicinal plants and identified a number of substances (some narcotics) including quinine and morphine. During this period a fairly familiar substance of our present day was also discovered, 'caffeine'.

Although in this new era chemists/scientists were able to investigate and research more plants in a real scientific way, the tendency was growing to isolate the active principals of plants. This led to the replacement of the use of a great number of essential oils by synthetic substances, many have indeed been very effective but against the success has to be measured the side effects of some.

Renée Gattefossé

THE 20TH CENTURY

Essential oils continued to be used by the pharmaceutical industry into the present century. A small number are still in use today: ; Lavender, Peppermint and Myrrh. Until the 20th century essential oils had been classified along with herbal remedies and cosmetics.

Our modern knowledge of aromatherapy stems from the early 1920's. Although progress with research and discoveries was slow and somewhat random, William Minchin, the English Doctor, discovered the benefits of garlic oil and had great success in treating patients with T.B. and diphtheria. The Italian doctors Giovanni Gatti and Renato Cayola were working on the psycotherapeutic applications of essential oils. The Australian Doctor Penfold was working with Tea-Tree oil. Research was also taking place in the USA, Japan and the USSR.

It was a French cosmetic chemist, Renée Gattefosse who coined the term 'Aromatherapie' in 1937. Gattefosse is looked on as the father of aromatherapy; his interests were in the anti-microbial effects of the oils and in their application to the skin for both cosmetic and medicinal purposes. He published both a scientific paper and book. His personal interest in the use of Lavender oil for the treatment of burns was aroused following an accident in the laboratory in which he badly burned his hand. To ease the pain he put his hand into the nearest bowl of essential oil; this happened to be lavender. The burn healed quickly leaving no trace of a scar. He continued his research into essential oils publishing a book entitled 'Aromatherapie'.

The progress of aromatherapy came almost to a standstill with the second world war. The notable exception being Dr Jean Valnet. He had been influenced by the work of

Gattefosse and was using essential oils as antiseptics when treating soldiers. After the war he continued to use the oils; he also taught other doctors how to use the oils. Today there are numerous doctors in France using essential oils and many fine training establishments where medical doctors can learn the art.

France was to give the next great aromatherapist of our time a chance to explore and work with the oils in a much wider field. Marguerite Maury, born in Austria, had a great love for botany and biochemistry. She married at a very early age and after a number of tragic incidents in her life she qualified as a nurse and surgical assistant. She moved to France where she worked for many years as a nursing assistant to a surgeon in Alsace. It was while there that she was given a book which had been written by Dr Chabenes, published in 1838 (the author later taught Dr. Gattefosse). The book became Marguerite's bible. She dedicated her life to aromatherapy and tried to prove the value of essential oil on the wellbeing of people. She lectured and gave seminars on the subject in France, Switzerland and England. Marguerite Maury ran courses for, and lectured to, Beauty Therapists who during the sixties became the first Aromatherapists in England. After just one or two years the practice of including Aromatherapy as part of the training in Beauty Therapy stopped. It became no longer necessary for the Beauty Therapist to learn about the individual oils he/she could purchase and use. The therapist began to use pre-blended oils in massage; this is a practice which continues today and has led to confusion amongst members of the public.

A qualified Aromatherapist will be recognised by one or more of the major professional bodies such as I.F.A. or I.S.P.A.. Details of these organisations are available at the end of this book

BASIC BIOLOGY OF PLANTS AND FLOWERS

Plants and animals, including man, owe their existence to the presence of a complicated chemical substance known as Deoxyribonucleic Acid or DNA for short. This material contains the genes and controls the activities of the organism. Life is literally dependent on the presence of this DNA. Plants are similar to man in other ways, not least in that there are substantial areas of function that are not completely understood.

The basic units from which plants develop are called cells. These exist in a wide variety of shapes and forms, each type specialised to carry out a particular function. Each cells length, width and thickness is regulated by chemical reaction. The growth of a whole plant involves the growth of roots, stems, leaves, flowers and other structures. For a healthy plant to grow there has to be a continuous supply of new cells to add to those already in existence. The supply of these new cells is achieved by a process of cell division. In the later life of the plant, when the roots and stems begin to thicken (a process known as secondary thickening), there is further cell division.

THE ROOT OF THE PLANT

The root of the plant performs two important functions in the life of the plant.

1. It provides firm support for the rest of the plant by anchoring these roots firmly to the ground.

2. The roots extract water and dissolved nutrients from the soil.

STEMS

The main function of the stem is:-

1.   To provide support for the leaves and flowers in such a way as they can best absorb sunlight.

2.   To provide a transport system for the distribution of substances within the plant.

LEAVES

The function of a leaf is almost always the same whatever the shape. That function is the production of energy. The cells of a leaf contain pigment (a coloured substance) the most important being chlorophyll which absorbs light from the sun's rays. This is converted into a form of energy and the energy used to power a series of reactions, a process which is known as Photosynthesis (because it depends on light). During this process plants take in carbon dioxide directly from the air. It enters the leaf through minute pores called stoma found on the surface of the leaf. Oxygen is a by-product of photosynthesis. Put simply, molecules of water are split into the two elements, hydrogen and oxygen, of which they are composed. Some of the oxygen is used by the plant, the remainder is released into the air. The hydrogen combines with the carbon, from carbon-dioxide to form various kinds of plant sugars which are called carbohydrates. Without photosynthesis the human race could not survive as there would be nothing to eat. This must surely make photosynthesis one of the most important processes on earth.

LEAF TYPES

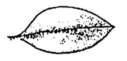

Simple

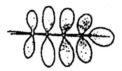

Pinnate

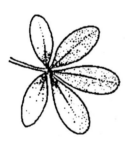

Palmate

LEAF MARGINS

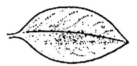

Entire

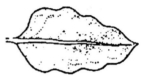

Undulated

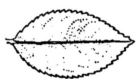

Dentate

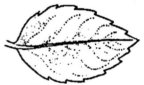

Serrate

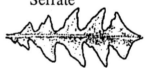

Pinnatisect

LEAF SHAPES

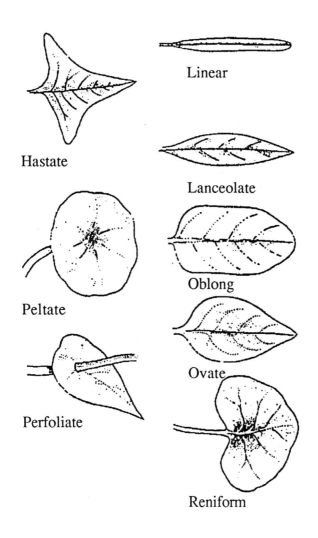

Hastate

Linear

Lanceolate

Peltate

Oblong

Perfoliate

Ovate

Reniform

LEAF ARRANGEMENTS

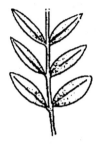

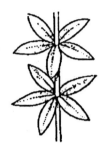

| Opposite | Alternate | Whorled |

LEAF TIPS

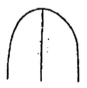

| Acute | Acuminate | Blunt |

FLOWERS

Flowers are believed by most people to be the most beautiful and interesting part of a plant. Flowers are arranged in spirals or whorls around a central stalk. Flowers consist of four component parts:-

1. **Sepals.** They look like tiny leaves and are collectively known as calyx. Their function is mainly protective.

2. **Petals.** These are found just inside the sepals. In some flowers the sepals and the flowers are not very distinct. The petals are normally brightly coloured in order to attract insects, which is important for the process of pollination and the life cycle of the plant.

3. **Stamen.** This is the male reproductive part of the flower found in the centre of the flower. The stamen consists of a slender stalk called a filament, which ends in a sack-like structure called Anthers. It is inside the anthers that thousands of pollen grains are produced. These pollen grains contain the male sex cell, or gamete, which can fertilise a female egg cell.

4. **Pistil.** This is the female reproductive part of the plant found in the centre of the flower, The pistil consists of a protective structure called the Ovary or Carpel. This contains one or more ovules, one or more female egg cell is contained in each ovule. At the top of the ovary is a slender projection called the style; this ends in a specialised pollen receiving region known as the Stigma. For fertilisation to take place the male sex cell (a pollen grain) must become attached to the stigma. It then germinates to produce a pollen tube which grows through the style to reach the ovule. The male and female sex cells fuse and an embryo is formed, which may grow into a new plant.

Note! Not all plants contain both the male and female reproductive parts.

POLLINATION

In self-pollination plant grains are transported from the anthers to stigma on the same individual plant, whereas in cross-pollination plant pollen is transferred to the stigmas of different individuals of the same species.

INFLORESCENCE

The way flowers can be grouped together in arrangements is called inflorescence and this can be important in identifying flowers.

Some of the common types of inflorescence are:-

Spike, Raceme, Panicle, Cyme, Umbel, Capitulum.

FLOWER STYLES

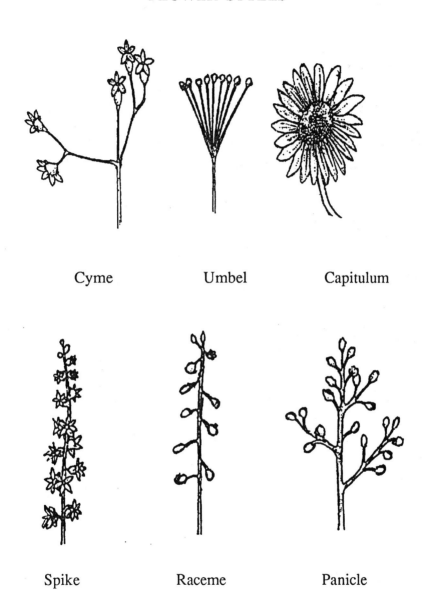

Cyme   Umbel   Capitulum

Spike   Raceme   Panicle

PLANT MATERIAL

There are various systems for classifying plant material. The most common is the Organographic System. This classifies the plant's raw material according to the part of the plant gathered.

From - the part of the plant below ground (Subterranean):

Bulb	Bulbus
Rhizome	Rhizoma
Root	Radix
Tuber	

From - the part of the plant above ground :

Bark	Cortex
Bud	Gemma
Fruit	Fructus
Flower	Flos
Glands	Glandulae
Herb	Herba
Leaf	Folium
Seed	Stamen
Stalk	Caulis
Stripe	Stipes

CLASSIFICATION OF PLANTS

Through his books *Genera Plantarum* and *Critica Botanica*
published in 1737, the great Swedish botanist Carl Von Linné,
usually known as Carl Linnaeus, formalised a new scientific
language - Botanical Latin. In this language each species was
given a two part latin name (binomial). This name was unique
and separated the name and description.

The first part of the Latin name denotes the genus and may be
shared by many other species. The second part either
commemorates a famous botanist (often the person who
discovered it) or refers to some feature of the species.

Linnaeus based his botanical classification on the number of
carpels and stamens. This was an artificial system which led
to some anomalies. Through time and in the light of new
knowledge small parts of his original works were revised,
though most of the genera he classified still remains the same. ·

In spite of the general acceptance internationally of the rules of
nomenclature, plants have been named and described by a
number of different people which can still sometimes cause
confusion. A great number of botanical names are still followed
by the suffix 'L' . A tribute to his accuracy.

I have attempted to put the more commonly used oils into their
botanical headings.

ANNONANCEAE

Over 2,000 species make up this almost entirely tropical family of trees and shrubs. In the Tropics various species are used for medicine, ointment and perfume.

OILS OF THIS FAMILY :

Ylang-Ylang

BURSERACEAE

A plant of the desert and tropics credited with anti-inflammatory powers .

OILS OF THIS FAMILY:

Frankincense
Myrrh

COMPOSITAE

The largest botanical family, these plants grow mainly in open spaces in most parts of the world. The exceptions being the tropical forests and the most northerly regions.
Credited with a great diversity of healing powers.

OILS OF THIS FAMILY:

Chamomile German
Chamomile Roman

CONIFERAE/CUPRESACEAE

The name Conifer implies a tree that bears cones and needles. The oldest and highest trees of the world found in both Northern and Southern hemispheres. Fom this family come many producers of paper and wood pulp as well as essential oils

OILS OF THIS FAMILY:

Juniper
Cypress

GERANIACEAE

Geranium. The plant of strong adaptability. Geranium Robertianum is the wild geranium found in various parts of the temperate world. It is totally different to the types used for the extraction of oils; namely Pelargonium Graveolens and Pelargonium Odrantissimum (rose scented).

OILS OF THIS FAMILY :

Geranium

GRAMINEAE

The nutritious plants of the earth; its intricate network of roots blending with the soil. Graminae include not only the common grasses but also barley, corn, oats, rice and wheat as well as the tropical spices.

Oils of this Family:

Lemongrass
Citronella
Palma Rosa.

LABIATAE

The plants associated with curative powers. They are found
in open spaces in moderate climates.

Oils of this Family:

Basil	Clary-Sage
Lavender	Marjoram
Melissa	Patchouli
Peppermint	Rosemary
Spearmint	Thyme

MYRTACEAE

The plant of harmony. It grows mainly in the tropics.

Oils of this Family :

Cajuput
Eucalyptus
Niaouli
Tea-Tree

OLEACEAE

Shrubs and tree of the sub tropical or temperate climates. The name Jasmine is derived from the Persian Yasmin. It belongs to the genus Jasminum from the family Oleaceae

OILS OF THIS FAMILY:

Jasmine	Grandiflorum	Essential Oil
Jasmine	Officinale	Essential oil
Jasmine	Sambac	Scenting Tea
Jasmine	Panticulatum	(China) Scenting Tea

PIPERACEAE

About 1,000 species into 10 genera. Distributed throughout the tropics. Used in medicine, food and beverages.

OILS OF THIS FAMILY:

Black Pepper

ROSACEAE

3000 or more species in 100 genera of the Rose family.

OILS OF THIS FAMILY:

Rose

RUTACEAE

Plants/trees of this Rue family number more than sixteen hundred, grouped into about 150 genera. They are found in tropical, subtropical and temperate regions.
The oils produced by this family are refreshing and cooling. It has been known for some handlers of the essential oils from the Rutaceae family to develop dermatitis.

OILS OF THIS FAMILY:

Bergamot	Mandarin
Grapefruit	Neroli
Lemon	Orange
Lime	Petitgrain
Tangerine	

SANTALACEAE

The Sandalwood family of shrubs and trees all of semiparasitic nature and consisting of some 400 species grouped into 30 genera. This family is found in tropical and temperate regions.

OILS OF THIS FAMILY:

Sandalwood

STYRACEAE

About 175 species of trees and shrubs grouped into twelve genera. Widely distributed, some species produce aromatic resins.

OILS OF THIS FAMILY:

Benzoin

UMBELLIFERAE

A family of 3,000 species in about 300 genera. Found mainly in the temperate zones of the northern hemisphere with a considerable number occurring wild in the USA

OILS OF THIS FAMILY:

Fennel Sweet

ZINGIBERACEAE

Ginger (Zingiber Officinale) noted for its medicinal properties and used for thousands of years in China and India.

OILS OF THIS FAMILY :

Ginger

HOW ARE THE OILS EXTRACTED FROM THE PLANTS?

Essential oil is produced by:-

1.	Distillation:	Water or Steam
2.	Expression:	Sponge
3.	Ecuelle:	Barrel/Spikes
4.	Maceration:	Hot Fat
5.	Extraction:	Enfleurage or Solvent
6.	Solvent:	Absolute

DISTILLATION

The most common method used to obtain the oils is steam distillation. In this method the plant is held in a container above boiling water. The steam produced by the water draws off the essential oil. The oil and steam travel to a further collecting chamber where the steam is cooled to form water in which the essential oil will either sink to the bottom or float to the top depending on its density. The water is then drawn off leaving only the essential oil.

ENFLEURAGE

The procedure for obtaining essential oil by the enfleurage method is extremely labour intensive and no longer widely used.

Chassis, the name given to the wooden framed glass (much like small windows in appearance) are prepared by coating the glass with a film of specially purified fat. Freshly picked flowers are placed on to the layers of fat and the chassis are then stacked one above the other. After some time (between 24 and 70 hours) the wilted flowers are removed and more fresh flowers are added to the enfleurage.

The enfleurage (fat mixture) becomes saturated with essential oil and is now called **pomade** (this product can be used as an ointment or perfume).

The **pomade** is then mixed with alcohol. The essential oil dissolves but the fat is insoluble in the alcohol and is drained off. The next step is to gently heat the alcohol so it evaporates, leaving the essential oil in the container.

EXPRESSION

This method is reserved for citrus fruits. The rind is grated or squeezed into a sponge and when the sponge becomes saturated the oil is squeezed into a container. Since the 1930's machines have taken over from man for this process. The workers involved in handling the sponges full of essential oils used to suffer quite severe allergic reactions especially on the hands. Hence this is one area where the machine is welcomed to take over the job of man.

EUCELL

This was a traditional method of obtaining the oils from the citrus family. Revolving barrel-type drums lined with spikes were packed with citrus fruits. The movement jarred the fruit against the spikes puncturing it and releasing the oil to be drained off and stored.

MACERATION

This is a similar method to enfleurage. The part of the plant to be used is plunged into hot fat which penetrates the cells of the plant, absorbing their oils. When the fat is saturated the process to collect the essential oil is then performed. This process is the same as that performed in the second stage of enfleurage. It should be noted that in this method the plant is sometimes crushed or broken up prior to or during the process of obtaining the oil.

SOLVENT

Solvent extraction is a complicated process. The flowers, gums or resins are placed in a container and covered with a solvent (Acetone or any petroleum by-product) to extract the oil. This is followed by various heating, cooling and filtering processes which results in a dark coloured paste known as concrete. To obtain an absolute from the concrete alcohol is added; into which a number of the constituents dissolve. The alcohol is then evaporated off completely and the resulting mix is known as an **Absolute.**

DEFINITION OF SOME TERMS USED IN EXTRACTION

Concrete:
During the solvent extraction process prior to the addition of alcohol the solvents are evaporated off, leaving behind a dark coloured paste known as concrete which contains both natural waxes, odiferous molecules and some chemical residue. Concrete should never be used for aromatherapy treatments as it contains chemical residue from the solvents.

Resiniod:
Prepared from dead organic material benzoin, frankincense and myrrh. Gums and resins are immersed in acetone in which they dissolve. The acetone is then evaporated off and the remaining heavy sticky substance is known as a Resinoid (or Resin Absolute). Resinoids are used mainly by the perfumery industry as fixatives.

An oil can be obtained from both Frankincense and Myrrh by steam distillation.

Benzoin is unsuitable for steam distillation as it is insufficiently volatile.

Pomades:
Pomades are the oil laden fat products of a process known as Enfleurage.

WHAT ARE THE OILS MADE OF?

Each essential oil is made up of numerous different organic molecules. The aromatic and therapeutic properties of each essential oil depends on the combination and concentration of these molecules which belong to several different chemical families including the following:-
Acids, Alcohols, Aldehydes, Esters, Ketones, Phenols and Terpenes, and many more including some still to be discovered; in fact chemists are still unable to reconstitute some essential oils with complete accuracy. It should be noted that the plant's genetic make-up dictates the final composition of the essence.

Any variation due to weather conditions, the time of day or night the plant has been harvested, the soil and altitude in which the plant has been grown will all cause some variations. As with wines there can be good and bad years, but of course the oil or essence should always be recognisable as being that of the plant to which it is specific.

Although technically we are using oils, **essential oils** are different from all other types of oil. They are not a fatty substance. This can be demonstrated by dropping a globule of the oil on to a plain piece of paper. The oil will evaporate leaving no oil mark on the paper.

Essential oil is not readily soluble in water but is soluble in alcohol, vegetable and mineral oil.

Essential oils are:
Volatile, flammable and odoriferous

CHEMICAL CONSTITUENTS OF ESSENTIAL OIL

The chemical constituents of essential oils are determined by two factors:

1. Intrinsic factors (occurring within the plant)

These are the internal processes in the plant cells that make each individual type of plant produce a different range of end products from simple hydrogen and carbon building blocks. The way in which the building blocks are able to combine in different permutations is determined by the genetic make up of each plant type.

2. Intrinsic factors (occurring outside the plant)

Many factors can introduce subtle changes in the combination of individual constituents. The growing conditions of the plant, i.e. soil type, climate, harvesting processes, should be considered. By far the greatest factor is the extraction process by which the oil is obtained. The action of heat and steam in the distillation process creates chemicals in the essential oils that are not present naturally in the living plants.

One important fact which should be remembered by all therapists is that one of the special characteristics of essential oil molecules is that their size is very small and it is this fact that enables the essential oil to penetrate the skin.

From a therapeutic point of view the following classifications
of constituents of essential oils may be found to be most
useful :

TERPENES (SUFFIXED - ENE)

Terpenes are hydrocarbons consisting of hydrogen and carbon
atoms. They are unsaturated molecules (i.e. contain one or
more carbon/carbon double bonds) which allows them to
react easily with oxygen to produce the terpenoids. Three
classes of terpenes are found in essential oils.

MONOTERPENES (MONOCYCLIC, BICYCLIC)

These have a 10 carbon atom backbone. They are small
enough to distil with steam and they are the main constituents
of many essential oils. Monoterpenes such as Limonene and
Pinene, have antiviral and antiseptic properties respectively.

SESQUITERPENES

These have a 15 atom backbone and are also commonly found
molecules in essential oils. In spite of being less volative than
the monoterpenes they can still be distilled with steam.
Essential oils with a high proportion of sesquiterpene
constituents are mostly distilled from roots and woods or
from plants of the Asteraceae family. Chamomile oil
contains Chamazulene and the sesquiterpenoid - Farnesol,
both of which have anti-inflammatory and antibacterial
properties.

DITERPENES

These have 20 carbon atoms, are less common in essential oils
and not readily steam distilled

OXYGENATED DERIVATIVES:
The most common are oxygen derivatives of terpenes :

ALDEHYDES - (SUFFIXED - AL OR ALDEHYDE)

The monoterpenoid alderhydes Citral and Citronellal are the
principal chemical features of such oils as Melissa and
Citronella. Many examples have sedative and/or antiseptic
properties. Structurally the oxygen is attached to a carbon
linked to a hydrogen and the functional group is located at the
end of a carbonic chain.

KETONES - (SUFFIXED - ONE)

This functional group is produced by the attachment of an
oxygen atom to a carbon atom within the carbonic chain.
Ketones are among the most toxic constituents found in
essential oils. They are found in Woodworm, Sage and Tansy;
and Pulegone, found in Pennyroyal, is particularly hazardous.
Not all ketones are toxic and the therapist needs to look at
them carefully.

ESTERS - (SUFFIXED - ATE)

The ester functional group contains 2 oxygen atoms. The
second oxygen atom is bonded to the carbon of the carboxyl
group. Esters are produced through the reaction of an alcohol
with an acid, i.e. Lanalool + Acetic acid = Linalyl Acetate
(principal ester in Lavender, Clary Sage) + Water. Esters are
among the most widespread group found in essentrial oils and
both have sedative and fungicidal properties. They provide
the finer notes to many fragrances

ALCOHOLS - (SUFFIXED - OL OR ALCOHOL)

Oxygen is attached to the carbon atom of the parent molecule through a single bond in the hydroxyl group, in which hydrogen takes up the second bond. These are among the most useful group of compounds. They are generally non-toxic and are uplifting with antiviral and antisceptic qualities.

PHENOLS - (ALSO SUFFIXED - OL)

Structurally, in this group, the hydroxyl group is attached to a benzene ring. Thymol and Carvacrol, found in Thyme, are very strong antibacterials and in common with other phenols, have strong stimulating effects. They should be used only in appropriately low concentrations as they can cause skin irritation.

OXIDES

The most important oxide is Eucalyptol (Cineol) which is the principal constituent of Eucalyptus oil. It is found to a lesser degree in Rosemary, Tea-Tree and Cajuput and has a strong expectorant effect.

PHENYLPROPANES

These compounds have a phenyl ring system with a propane (three carbon atom) side chain. This (nine carbon atom) structure can be modified by various functional groups added to it, as in the terpenes. The special electron configuration in these structures allows some pharmacologically highly active molecules to be produced. Like the phenols Cinnamic aldehyde and Eugenol (found in Cinnamon and Clove respectively), they are very strong antiseptics but used in excess can cause severe skin reactions. Other examples such as Methyl Chavicol and Myristicin (Nutmeg), can cause negative effects if used in unreasonably high concentrations.

Other molecules occur in plants but do not find their way to the essential oil. The reason for their absence is that their molecule size or weight is too high to evaporate with steam.

NOTE
The suffixes quoted above are only a guide to the constituents group e.g. not all Ketones are suffixed -ONE and not all Phenols are suffixed -OL etc....

ARE ALL ESSENTIAL OILS SAFE TO USE?

Generally speaking essential oils are beneficial. However, it is not a truism to say because it is natural it is safe. Essential oils should always be used with care and caution! Some essential oils are highly toxic and should never be used. All professional aromatherapists should know this list of oils. Anyone considering using essential oils should firstly check with a qualified therapist.

Some essential oils if used in too high a dosage can induce, for example, giddiness in people who have a tendency towards this condition. Some essential oils can be toxic, having harmful effects if used over a long period of time. It is a good idea to take a break from the daily use of the same oils at six weekly intervals.

A period of at least twenty-four hours should be allowed to elapse between each full body massage. I believe two full Aromatherapy body massages per week to be sufficient.

As previously mentioned, certain oils should never be used for any conditions. In the interest of safety the therapist must also familiarise him/herself with the side effects of particular oils and when and where they must not be used.

Great care should be taken with pregnant women, children, the elderly; also those suffering with serious illnesses, contagious conditions, allergies, asthma, hayfever, rhinitis, sensitive skins epilepsy or diabetes; a number of oils are not recommended in these circumstances. Constant referral to text books and knowledge up-dated through professional therapists/ organisations is a must for all who use essential oils.

SAFETY AND PRECAUTIONS

FIRE

Essential oils are flammable and should be kept away from naked flames. Materials (for example: couch roll or tissues used to mop up spillage of essential oils) should be put into an external waste bin. This material should not be put into the usual waste bins/area inside the work place. There is always the danger of a match, cigarette or hot candle being thrown into the bin or it being left near a source of heat.

ESSENTIAL OILS INTERNALLY

No essential oil should be taken by mouth (internally) unless prescribed by a medically qualified **doctor**. If essential oil is taken internally by accident then seek medical advice.

SPLASHES OF ESSENTIAL OIL INTO THE EYE

The eye should be washed immediately and bathed with lots of water; use an eye-bath if possible and change the water repeatedly. If the eye feels sore or continues to be painful get medical help.

SPLASHES OF ESSENTIAL OIL INTO THE MOUTH

Rinse the mouth out several times with water. If the inside of the mouth feels sore or painful seek medical advice. However, in most cases the latter step will not be necessary.

SPLASHES OF ESSENTIAL OIL ON THE SKIN

Wash the area thoroughly. Normally this course of action should prevent any adverse reaction but obviously it will depend on the oil being used and the amount splashed on the skin.

SAFETY AND STORAGE

Always keep essential oils out of the reach of children. Use a locked cabinet or locked refrigerator. Do not leave oils in a normal household refrigerator where there is a danger of them being used by mistake.

LABELLING

Make sure all bottles are clearly labelled (use a well gummed label). Clearly type or use a good indelible pen. Include the following information;

1. Date   2. Base oil   3. Essential oil used (a professional therapist would normally use the botanical name)

4. Name and telephone number of the person who blended the oil

5. Instructions for use

SPECIFIC TO THE PROFESSIONAL THERAPIST

The professional therapist will need to label the bottle of the blended oils(s); it is also advisable that he/she keep a separate Sales Book. Record the following information :
Client's name
Address
Telephone number
Date
Condition/Symptom
Instructions given for home use
Total quantity of oil sold (e.g. 50ml)
Base and essential oil used including percentage
Amount charged for each preparation

If you keep a stock of oils then it is a wise precaution to speak with your supplier about fire regulations and storage.

METHODS OF USING ESSENTIAL OILS IN AROMATHERAPY

MASSAGE

Massage is probably the most important and useful way to use essential oils in aromatherapy and all the benefits of massage are difficult to measure. The oils work on the emotional as well as the physical plane (when absorbed through the skin). The inter-relation between mind and body in massage is one of the main keys to its importance. Physical massage relaxes not only muscles and improves lymph and blood flow, it also helps to relieve tension and balance the body's energy flow. It promotes a feeling of well being and aids the absorption of oils into the skin. Aromatherapy massage should be considered to be a truly holistic therapy treating mind and body.

Each therapist has his/her own routine for massage. The variety of techniques is enormous but it really does not matter which method is used providing the therapist has had a really thorough training. Most importantly the massage should physically encompass the whole body as the therapist takes into consideration the whole person body and mind. Massage provides the therapist with the most effective way of introducing the oils into the body.

Massage improves lymph and blood flow thus bringing oxygen and nutrients to the tissues and removing waste products of cell metabolism.

COMPRESSES

This is a very simple way of using essential oils especially when massage is contra-indicated or if treating a specific condition such as a sprain, bruising, menstrual camp or rheumatism.

Method:

Prepare a container of either hot or cold water. Add to this the required amount of the chosen oil; soak a clean cloth in the preparation and then wring out the excess water. The cloth is then put on the area to be treated. Maximum benefit is gained by repeatedly soaking and wringing out the cloth and putting it on the affected area. **Hot compresses** are often used in chronic conditions, menstrual cramp and headaches caused through tension, especially if the back of the neck seems to be affected. **Cold compresses** seem to be more effective for reducing swelling and relieving pain; they can also be effective for some headaches.

Compresses can be used in almost any area as it is easy to mould the material to the contours of the body including the face.

BATHS

The majority of essential oils are not absorbed by water; the droplets stay on the top of the water. The benefits are gained by breathing in the odoriferous molecules which are produced. By blending the oils in a carrier and then applying them to the bath the beneficial effects are three-fold; a. by osmosis through the skin to the bloodstream, b. through breathing and c. there is less danger of a reaction to the oil if used correctly. If undiluted oils are used in the bath then no more than four drops should be used in the average bath. If the oil is a blended oil then up to a maximum of 3 teaspoons (=15 ml) may be used. No oil should ever be used in the bath without first checking its properties, as some oil can be an irritant to the skin. If there is any doubt about skin sensitivity or allergies then test the oil in much lower quantities first and gradually increase the drops to the recommended amount. In order to gain maximum benefit from the bath it is best to stay in the bath at least fifteen minutes; twenty minutes being an ideal length of time to soak. Cool baths are invigorating, while hot baths have a calming effect. Very hot baths should be avoided, especially in cases of cardio vascular conditions, during pregnancy and by those who are not physically very active. Hot baths are also very drying on the skin.

INHALATION OR STEAMING

Inhalation is an old remedy for colds and flu. It is another simple way to use the oils for a specific purpose ranging from chest to skin problems. Place two to three drops of pure essential oil in a bowl of boiling water (when using a blended oil then the quantity can be doubled). Lean over the bowl with a large towel enclosing both your head and the bowl and inhale. The face should be about ten inches from the water and make sure to come out from under the towel every few minutes. Begin with about **half a minute** under the towel gradually building up to a few minutes. Breathing through the mouth helps sore throats, while breathing through the nose helps to unblock nasal passages. Once again, as with the bath oil, the properties of the oil should be checked. This treatment is sometimes offered by the professional therapist instead of, or prior to, another treatment; for example a facial massage, especially to clients suffering with sinusitis. **Note :** If you have sensitive skin especially with high pink/red colour or obvious thread veins the first thing to do, before preparing the inhalation is to cover the face in a thick layer of moisturiser or ointment base. Ideally this would be non-perfumed. It is also important to remember to close your eyes immediately you go under the towel.

VAPORISATION

The benefits and methods of evaporating essential oils seem endless. From placing a damp cloth, previously soaked in oil/water, on the radiator to burning the oils in special burners or on ingeniously designed rings which fit onto lamp bulbs and containers that fit onto radiators. Oils used in this way can vary from Tea-tree or Eucalyptus for 'flu bouts' to relaxing oils like Marjoram or Ylang-Ylang, Lavender and Chamomile through to 'wake me up' oils such as Rosemary and Peppermint. If using oils in the home then do consider the feelings of all the household. Do they all share the same needs?

ABSORPTION OF OILS

The molecular structure of the oil is very small, therefore it can be absorbed through the different layers of the skin and into the blood stream. When essential oil molecules evaporate into the air they can be taken down into the lungs along with the air we breathe. Some will be exhaled in the next breath but some will pass, as oxygen does, into the bloodstream and travel around the body. As far as we know essential oils do not remain in the body but are passed out in exhalation, perspiration, urine and faeces. Expulsion usually takes three to seven hours in the average healthy body and up to fourteen hours in the obese. Some books and therapists recommend essential oil to be taken by mouth. I, however, believe that **no essential oil should be taken orally unless prescribed by a medically qualified and recognised doctor**; not only is the absorption of the oil through the skin safer it must surely be quicker than when the oil is trying to cope with the complex workings of the digestive system and the sensitive mucous membranes it encounters on its journey.

OILS - CARRIER OR BASE ?

Carrier oils are also known as Base Oils. Essential oils are mixed (blended) in a carrier oil before application to the skin.

In the following pages I will endeavour to give some background information that should help decision making with regard to the most suitable carrier oil to use for a specific purpose.

NOTE

Ethol Alcohol is sometimes used as a carrier (i.e. Verruca treatment or perfume base.) I have chosen to suggest Vodka as a carrier for some of my recipes as it is more readily available for home use. The professional therapist will normally use Ethol Alcohol.

CARRIER OILS

ALMOND OIL (SWEET)

Skin   Dry, itching, inflamed,
                            sensitive.
                            It is obtained from the
                            kernel

Contains   Minerals, vitamins,
                            proteins and glucosides

Colour   Pale yellow

APRICOT KERNEL

Skin   Dry, dehydrated, inflamed
                            or mature. It is obtained
                            from the kernel

Contains   Minerals and vitamins

Colour   Pale Yellow

CORN OIL

Skin   All skin types

Contains   Proteins, vitamins and
                            minerals

Colour   Pale yellow

GRAPESEED OIL

Skin

All skin types. Very light, almost odourless, therefore does not interfere with the aroma of the essential oil. It is also one of the least expensive carrier, base oils

Contains

Vitamins, proteins and minerals

Colour

Pale green to colourless

HAZELNUT OIL

Skin

All skin types. This oil has a slight astringent action. It is obtained from the kernel.

Contains

Minerals, vitamins and proteins

Colour

Yellow

JOJOBA OIL

Skin

All skins. Penetrates easily. It is especially good for acne, eczema, inflamed skins and psoriasis. This oil can feel a little sticky owing to its waxy substance (mimics collagen). In view

of this latter substance
many therapists will use
the oil as a carrier for
facial treatment; its
penetrating powers makes
it a useful oil when treating
clients with a lot of
subcutaneous tissue (fat)

Contains   Minerals and proteins

Colour   Yellow

OLIVE OIL
Uses   Mainly when rheumatic
                                   conditions are present and
                                   as a nourishing treatment for
                                   the hair. Disadvantage - it
                                   has a strong smell which is
                                   difficult to disguise

Contains   Minerals, vitamins and
                                   proteins

Colour   Green

SESAME OIL

Skin	Eczema, psoriasis. Other uses- arthritis, rheumatism, general aches and pains. Advantage - this oil washes out of clothing fairly easily so indirectly could be considered the cheapest oil of all
Contains	Amino-acids, lecithin, minerals and vitamins
Colour	Dark yellow

PEANUT OIL, SOYABEAN OIL, SAFFLOWER OIL

Skin	All skin types
Contains	Minerals, vitamins and proteins
Colour	All three oils are pale yellow

SUNFLOWER OIL

Skin	All types
Contains	Minerals and vitamins (no proteins)
Colour	Pale yellow

OILS USED TO ENHANCE THE ACTION OF OTHER CARRIER OILS. USUALLY USED AS A 10% DILUTION

AVOCADO

Skin	Dry, dehydrated or eczema. Very good penetrating powers; can be blended with other oils when treating areas of fatty tissue. Avocado is considered amongst the best nourishing oils. It is seldom used on its own; this could have some bearing on the price, which is very high
Contains	Fatty acids, lecithin, proteins, and vitamins
Colour	Dark green

CARROT OIL

Skin	Dry, ageing, itching, eczema, psoriasis. It also helps to reduce scarring. Carrot oil is often added to creams for facial treatments. It should **not** be used on the skin in an undiluted form as there is a danger of turning the skin orange

Contains	Beta-carotene, minerals and vitamins
Colour	Orange

EVENING PRIMROSE OIL

In its natural state the evening primrose is a wild flower. It is the newest of the wild plants to be grown as a crop. Strictly speaking it is not a primrose at all but belongs to the willow herb family. Evening Primrose is a fixed oil not a volatile essence.

Skin	All skin types but particularly sensitive, psoriasis, eczema and itching. Other uses P.M.T., Menopause, Heart disease, M.S. and Rheumatoid Arthritis
Contains	Gamma linolic acid, minerals and vitamins
Colour	Pale yellow

Wheatgerm Oil

Skin	All types especially dry and prematurely ageing as well as for eczema and psoriasis. It is also an anti-scarring agent. **This oil is a natural anti-oxidant due to its vitamin E content; therefore 5% added to other carrier oils will prolong their shelf life.** As it is a very sticky oil it offers little lubrication therefore for use as a carrier it is best used in proportions of 25% wheatgerm to 75% of other base carrier oil
Contains	Minerals, proteins and vitamins
Colour	Yellow/Orange

CHOOSING THE CARRIER

The choice of carrier or base oil is governed by four main factors:

1. Smell
2. Texture
3. Price
4. Therapeutic value

In other words there should be little or no perfume. It should not be very sticky. It should give good slip and preferably not be very expensive. Grapeseed and Almond oil are the most popular. The heavier, richer oils, relatively speaking are :- Avocado, Jojoba and Wheatgerm.

Essential oils are nearly always blended before applying to the skin. There are only a few exceptions to this rule; Lavender being one of them as used in the treatment of burns.

Note: - Wheatgerm oil should not be used when the recipient suffers from gluten intolerance (wheat allergy) often referred to as Coeliac disease. I prefer not to use wheatgerm on Candida suffers or those with fungal infections such as Athlete's foot.

Sweet Almond is best avoided when recipient is a diabetic.

BLENDING GUIDE

Blending code for essential oil therapy

5 ml equals 100 drops, approximately 1 teaspoon.
Therefore when blending essential oils the following guide
should be applied:

¼% = 1 drop essential oil in 20 ml (or 400 drops) carrier

½% = 1 drop essential oil in 10 ml (or 200 drops) carrier

1% = 1 drop essential oil in 5 ml (or 100 drops) carrier

2% = 2 drops essential oil in 5 ml (or 100 drops) carrier

2½%= 5 drops essential oil in 10 ml (or 200 drops) carrier

3% = 3 drops essential oil in 5 ml (or 100 drops) carrier

The drops can only be an approximate measure as drop size
will differ according to the dispenser and the viscosity of the oil
(for accuracy it is advisable to purchase a suitably marked
measurer).

To prepare an aromatherapy blend add the required number of
drops to a clean, dry, empty bottle and then add the carrier (oil,
alcohol, etc.). Put the cap on tightly. Wipe the bottle and label.
Slowly turn the bottle upside down and back five times. Store
in a cool place ready for use.

A therapist could prepare basic blends on a weekly or even fortnightly basis. This is easily done if the average massage blending at 2% or 2½% is adhered to.

He/she can prepare the commonly used oils in 50 ml bottles. The less commonly used oils in 25 ml bottles and the stronger or least used oils in 10 ml bottles.

If oils are being prepared in this way the therapist should take some measures to protect themselves from a build-up of oils:

1.   Wear protective clothing (overall)
2.   Wear polythene gloves
3.   Wear a face mask
4.   Wear protective eye wear - glasses or swimming goggles
5.   Wear a hat or head band to avoid having to push hair off the face (touching face with a gloved hand)
6.   If you wear glasses and feel the need to re-position them on your nose, push them up using the forearm, not the hand.

My personal experience as a result of a lapse in this procedure was a very severe reaction on the right side of my nose and cheek (I am right handed) which made it difficult, if not impossible for me to wear my glasses for about three weeks.

When making products (face creams/toners/moisturisers) for daily use it is wise to keep the amount of essential oil to minimum percentages; as a general guide this could be in the region of 0.005 percent. The amount of oil needed for a full body massage is 15-20 ml depending on the size of the body; 5 ml being the average for a back or 5 ml for face and neck.

It is unwise to be subjected daily to oils in skin products, baths/shower, vapourisers and massage. According to the well known saying 'You can have too much of a good thing'.

If buying a pre-blended oil from a retail outlet it would be a wise precaution to ask the following questions :

1. Date the oil was blended?

2. If oils are purchased pre-blended or blended on site?

3. Under what conditions the oils are stored?

4. What percentage of essential oil is contained in the carrier?

5. Remember during the purchase and sell on process essential oils often pass through several hands before ending up on the shop shelf. If in doubt buy well known brand names available direct from the supplier or chosen oulets.

6 Purchase date and storage details may also be queried on pure, non-blended essential oils.

NOTE : A number of the oils being sold for use in vaporisers are synthetic. They are not true essential oils or absolutes.

TOP, MIDDLE AND BASE NOTES
WHAT DO THEY MEAN?

To the more modern Aromatherapist the notes are merely a guide. The idea of classification in this manner is taken from the world of the perfumer and is taken to mean, in that context, a distinctive odour effect which can be identified and named. The idea was devised by a nineteenth century Italian Septimus Piesse. He compared odours with sounds. Scents, he said, appear to influence the olfactory nerves in certain definite degrees. There is, as it were, an octave of odours like an octave in music. Certain odours coincide like the keys of an instrument. To each note Piesse assigned a note of the musical scale and to each note he assigned the odour of a natural source: middle C, for example, corresponded to Camphor, and so on. He believed that in order to create a harmonious perfume the odours appearing in his listings should be blended together to correspond with a cord formed from the respective musical notes (this method of blending perfumes no longer applies).

In perfume the top note is the first to be observed, it is the most volatile and lasts only between 10-30 minutes gradually giving way to the middle (or heart) note, which is the main fragrance of the perfume. This mixture is maintained with the support of a mixture from low volatile base notes.

The base notes slow down the volatility rate of the top and middle notes (they "fix" other essences). Therefore they are always used in perfume for their staying power. Two of the most commonly used fixatives (base notes) are Sandalwood and Patchouli.

Oils have the same odour strength or volatility. Therefore when an essential oil evaporates we have a constantly changing composition which in turn gives a constantly changing odour. This change is hardly noticeable as we continually smell the odour.

The theory of blending essential oils by note does have its faults as not all experts are in agreement as to which oils are top, middle and base. Some oils will also change depending on the crop, season and country of origin.

In view of these differences in Perfumery and Aromatherapy many Aromatherapists ignore the old perfumers' method of blending oils.

The blending of oils is very much a matter of individual choice for the professional therapist who has spent a long training period studying chemical compositions and is able to draw on his/her own experiences and results which have been guided and overseen by a tutor. Following that guidance is the only choice for the trainee and inexperienced therapist.

BLENDING

Blending by note: Relaxation - middle or base notes
                              Uplifting - middle or top notes

Top note   Most volatile - fast acting
Middle note   Moderately volatile
Base note   Least volatile

What to do: 1. Add top note
                              2. Add base or middle note
                              3. Add a carrier -(use a 'fixed' oil e.g. Grapeseed) -not very volatile

EVAPORATION

Evaporation simply means the change from liquid or solid to vapour.

The evaporation of a solid to vapour without first melting is called sublimation: in other words the solid slowly disappears over a period of time.

A typical example of evaporation, as we have all observed, is the drying up of a puddle of water. It is worth noting that the evaporation of alcohol and of water takes place much faster than the evaporation of an essential oil.

VOLATILITY
This could be simply explained as:

1. The speed (rate) of evaporation

2. The time taken for the odour of an oil to become undetectable under controlled conditions

3. Essential oils readily disappear in the open air. They are volatile

SHELF LIFE OF ESSENTIAL OILS BLENDED AND UNBLENDED

Essential oils evaporate very readily. They are damaged by exposure to air, light, cold and heat; in fact any temperature extremes.

Oils, in theory, should last for years but the more often they are exposed to air by opening, the greater the chance of oxidation, which will reduce the therapeutic value of the oil. It is easy to tell an oil that is old, not only by its aroma but also in some cases by the colour change and the cloudy appearance.

The therapist should aim to use all oils within a one year period.

Once essential oils have been diluted/blended their shelf life is drastically reduced to four or five months. Their lifespan can be prolonged for a little longer by the addition of wheatgerm oil which has anti-oxidant properties; 5% is usually added for this purpose (don't forget when not to use wheatgerm - see page 64).

All essential oils and those blended in a carrier/base oil for future use should be stored in dark glass bottles and clearly labelled.

Note - Wheatgerm oil tends to stain towels and couch covers.

PURCHASE AND STORAGE

Amber/brown bottles are ideal containers for the average person to use for the storage and transportation of essential oils. The amber/brown bottle protects the oil from the light which causes deterioration (Photcalatytic reaction). The screw cap should be kept tightly closed except when removing a quantity of oil for immediate use; this minimises the escape of essential oil vapour and the entry of air from the external atmosphere.

All aromatherapy oils should be stored in a cool place. Those of citrus and herb origin are best kept in a refrigerator (kept solely for the purpose of oil storage) at about 5 degrees Celsius. The wood oils keep pretty well at a constant room temperature of 15 degrees Celsius. The resinoids and gums will keep in a cool garage or basement.

Try to purchase oils in small quantities. If you are unlikely to use more than 10 ml of a particular oil every six months it is pointless to purchase 20 ml. If however, through circumstance it is necessary for you to purchase, for example, 20 ml at a time then perhaps it would be possible for you to share the cost and the quantity with a colleague. Divide the supply into four 5 ml bottles and label each bottle with:

1. The name of the oil - Botanical
2. The date of purchase
3. The supplier

Then take two bottles each. One for regular use and the other for storage. Alternatively keep three bottles in your cool dark storage area and bottle number four for your regular use.

Each time the bottle is opened some of the top note vapour will escape and at the same time air will get into the bottle bringing with it a new oxygen supply. By choosing and using the smallest sized bottle of essential oil, the amount of air in contact with the oil (in the bottle) is kept to a minimum, therefore helping to ensure the quality of the oil used.

When the essential oil bottle is empty or partly empty do not be tempted to refill this bottle with a fresh supply of oil as the fresh oil will become contaminated by the deteriorating dregs of the previous oil (some suppliers ask that their bottles be returned when empty).

I wash all my empty bottles in a solution of vinegar, Tea-Tree oil and salt, before placing them in the dishwasher. If you do not have a dishwasher then wash with suggested solution followed by a short (10 minute) soak in a solution of Epsom Salts (5 grams to 1 litre).

Note: Epsom Salts removes the oil smell from cloths, towels and dresses.

PURCHASE BOOK ENTRY

Date	Supplier	Product	Quantity	Cost	Comment
01.02.89	ML Gad	Jasmine	5 ml	£0	Kept
01.02.89	Hadwell	Tangerine	5 ml	£0	Returned - bad smell

CARRIAGE NOTES

Long Term

Today	Yester years
Glass bottles	Alabaster pots
Stainless Steel	Onyx pots
Aluminium	Wooden pots

Stainless steel drums with lacquered interiors are used in transportation and large quantity storage of esential oils.

Aluminium drums internally lacquered are used for storage and transportation of small amounts.

Plastic can be used for very short periods only as the oil will break down the plastic; hence there will be a detrimental effect on the essential oil.

It is important to note that the containers used for the storage of essential oils should be made of a material that will not allow air or light to the oil and will not cause any chemical interaction with the oil.

DIRECTORY OF SOME OF THE MORE COMMONLY USED ESSENTIAL OILS

BASIL

Note	Top
Botanical Name	Ocymum Basilicum
Family	Labiatae
Cultivation	France, (Asia, Mediterranean)
Part of Plant	Flowering tops and leaves
Extracted by	Steam Distillation
Yield 1 Gram Oil	Equals 2000 grams of base material
Constituents	**Terpenes** - Ocimene, Pinene, Sylvestrene. **Phenols** - Methylchavicol, Eugenol. **Ketones** - Borneone, Camphor. **Oxide** - Cineole. **Alcohol** - Linalool
Colour	Pale yellow
Aroma	Spicy
Blends well with	Geranium, Bergamot, Lavender, Clary-Sage, Sandalwood
Properties	Cephalic, Emmenagogue, Sudorific, Tonic

Most Common Uses

Respiratory

Chest infections, Asthma,
Bronchitis, Catarrh,
Hiccups, Whooping cough

Digestive

Indigestion,
Gastroenteritis, Vomiting

Head

Headaches, migraines, head
colds, mental fatigue,
insomnia (clears the mind)

Muscular

Tired, overworked muscles

Methods of use

Inhaler, Vapouriser,
Bath, Massage

Contra Indication

Pregnancy
Sensitive skins
Those prone to allergic
reactions

BASIL

An annual herb which grows to approximately 20cm in height.
The erect stems have numerous branches bearing opposite,
stalked, broadly ovate and pointed leaves. These leaves are
pale green in colour and bear purple ornaments.

The herb flowers in the summer producing white flowers
sometimes with a purple tinge.

Oil glands are dotted along the leaf.

My own use of this oil is not in massage or compress but in a
room burner when I need to keep a clear head and concentrate
on what is happening at the moment.

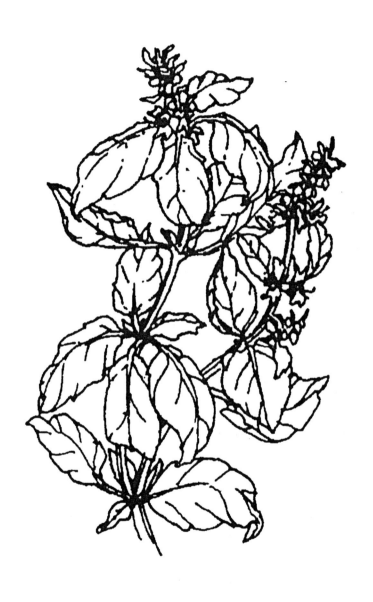

BASIL

BENZOIN

Note	Base
Botanical Name	Styrax Benzoin
Family	Styracaeeae
Cultivation	Java, Sumatra, Thailand
Part of Plant	Gum from tree
Extracted by	Steam distillation
Yield 1 Gram Oil	Equals 15 grams base material
Constituents	**Esters** - Benzyl benzoate. **Aldehydes** - Benzoic aldehyde (Benzaldehyde), Vanillin. **Acids** - Benzoic, Cinnamic.
Colour	Yellow/reddish brown
Aroma	Sweet, vanilla
Blends well with	Sandalwood, Rose, Jasmine
Properties	Antiseptic, Carminative, Deodorant, Diuretic, Expectorant, Sedative, Vulnerary

MOST COMMON USES

Respiratory	Bronchitis, Coughs, Asthma
Muscular - Joints	Arthritis, Rheumatism
Other	Gout, Colic, Sedative

CONTRA INDICATIONS	Children
Caution	May cause drowsiness, beware if operating machinery. Can be a skin sensitiser

BENZOIN

The Benzoin tree's main habitat is Java and Sumatra. This large tree grows to about 60 ft (20 m) in height. The leaves are pale green on top and whitish underneath. The tree does not produce Benzoin in the normal course of events. It is a pathological product obtained only after the infliction of a wound sufficiently severe to injure the bark and trunk. The tree then exudes or accumulates beneath the bark the liquid Benzoin. When the Benzoin hardens the tears (droplets) are collected.

The first incisions are made when the tree is seven years old. The tree continues to produce in this way for a further ten or so years. The finest quality being produced in the first three years. The final year's supply is obtained when the tree is felled and its contents scraped out.

My personal use of this oil is now in vapourisers. I no longer use it on the skin.

Most Common Uses

Respiratory   Bronchitis, Coughs,
                               Asthma

Muscular - Joints   Arthritis,   Rheumatism

Other   Gout, Colic, Sedative

Contra Indications   Children

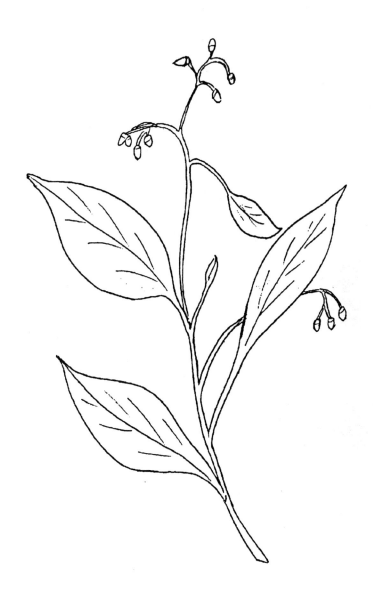

BENZOIN

BERGAMOT

Note	Top
Botanical Name	Citrus Bergamia
Family	Rutaceae
Cultivation	Italy, Morocco (West Africa)
Part of Plant	Rind of fruit
Extracted by	Expression
Yield 1 Gram Oil	Equals 200 grams ase material
Constituents	**Terpenes** - Dipentene, Limonene. **Lactone** - Bergaptene. **Ester** - Linalyl acetate. **Alcohols** - Linalool, Nerol, Terpineol
Colour	Green
Aroma	Citrussy, refreshing, light
Blends Well With	Cypress, Jasmine, Lavender, Neroli, Ylang-Ylang, Camomile, Marjoram
Properties	Analgesic, Antidepressant, Anti-Inflammatory, Antiseptic, Bactericide,

Deodorant, Expectorant,
Febrifuge, Sedative,
Vulnerary

Most Common Uses

Emotional

Tension/Anxiety,
Depression, Anorexia
Nervosa

Urinary

Urinary tract infections,
Urethritis, Cystitis, Vaginal
Pruritus

Skin

Acne, Infected, Oily

Other

Insect Repellent,
Deodorant, Personal and for
Rooms, Inhibits certain
viruses, Herpes Simplex,
Herpes Zoster (shingles),
Chickenpox

Methods of use

Bath, Compress, Massage,
Vapouriser

Contra Indications

Prior to, or immediatly
after, exposure to ultra
violet (Sun/Sunbed)

The chemical **Bergaptene** is responsible for increasing
photosensitivity of the skin. Bergaptene-free Bergamot is
available and does not effect the skin (do check oil and client
suitability).

BERGAMOT

The Bergamot tree grows to 15 feet (4.5m). The leaves are long and green, the flowers are white. The tree bears yellow, small, almost pear-shaped fruit. Harvest time is from December to February.

The main countries producing the oil are Italy and Sicily and to a lesser extent Africa. The oil has a long history and has been mentioned in many old herbals and manuscripts.

My favourite use for this beautiful green oil is in the room vapouriser. I tend not to use the oil on the skin in the summer months as skin reactions can occur when the skin is exposed to ultra violet light either from the sun or the use of a sunbed. In the winter months I do use the oil after warning my clients about U.V. exposure (Sun or Sunbeds).

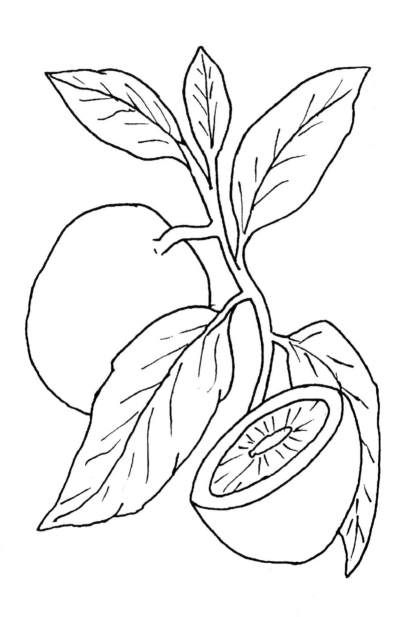

BERGAMOT

BLACK PEPPER

Note	Middle
Botanical Name	Piper Nigrum
Family	Piperaceae
Cultivation	Singapore, Sumatra, Penang, (East Asia)
Part of Plant	Unripe berries
Extracted by	Distillation
Yield 1 Gram Oil	Equals 50 grams base material
Constituents	**Sesquiterpene -** Caryophyllene, Bisabolene, Farnesene. **Terpenes -** Camphene, Limonene, Myrcene, Phellandrene, Pinene, Sabinene, Selinene, Thujene. **Phenols -** Eugenol, Myristicin, Safrole.
Colour	Colourless/palegreen/pale yellow
Aroma	Fresh peppercorns/warm
Blends Well With	Frankincense, Rosemary, Sandalwood, Marjoram, Lavender, Bergamot, Ylang-Ylang

Properties	Analgesic, Antiseptic, Antitoxic, Antispasmodic, Aphrodisiac, Carminative, Detoxicant, Febrifuge, Rubefacient, Diuretic, Digestive, Laxative, Stimulant, Stomachic, Tonic

MOST COMMON USES

Digestive	Colic, Indigestion, Constipation
Muscular	Aches, Pains, Rheumatic, Arthritic, Athletic aches and pains

METHODS OF USE	Compress, Local massage

CONTRA INDICATIONS	Can be a skin irritant

BLACK PEPPER

The Pepper is a native of Asia. In the cultivated state the
creeping vine grows to about 10-12ft (3-4m) in height but if left
untouched the vine can reach 20ft (6m) in height. Only at three
to four years old will the vine begin to produce peppers which
it will then continue to produce at the rate of about 4 lb. a year
for a further 15 years.

The leaves are dark green. The flowers small and white.

Pepper has been mentioned in many of the great scripts
throughout history; Chinese in the twelfth century,
Theophrastus and Pliny. Pepper was one of the spices that
inspired the voyages of exploration.

I find that to use this oil sparingly gives me good results
(I have only ever used it locally). My favourite uses for the oil
are: Muscular stiffness/fatigue prior to or directly after
running or dancing; also on local areas of rheumatic pain.

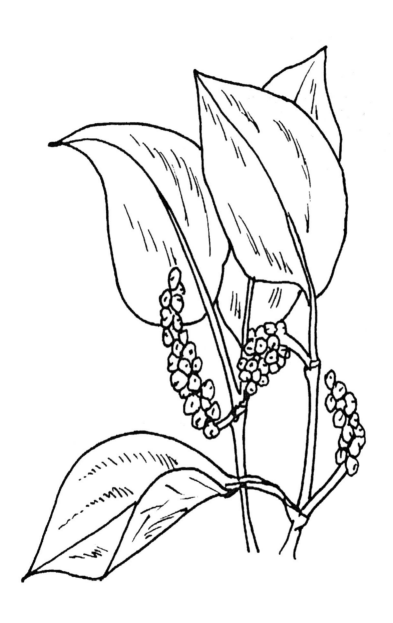

BLACK PEPPER

CAJUPUT

Note	Top
Botanical Name	Melaleuca Leucadendron
Family	Myrtaceae
Cultivation	Malaysia (Far East)
Part of Plant	Leaves/Buds
Extracted by	Steam distillation
Yield 1 Gram Oil	Equals 65 grams base material
Constituents	**Terpenes** - Pinene, Limonene, Dipentene. **Oxide** - Cineole. **Aldehyde** - Benzaldehyde. **Alcohol** - Terpineol
Colour	Pale yellow/pale green
Aroma	Camphorous
Blends Well With	Peppermint, Geranium, Lavender, Niaouli, Rose
Properties	Analgesic, Antineuralgic, Antirheumatic, Antiseptic Antispasmodic, Balsamic, Cicatrisant, Decongestant, Expectorant, Febrifuge, Insecticide, Stimulant, Sudorific

Most Common Uses

Respiratory System

Colds/Flu, Respiratory
Infections

Skin

Can be beneficial for some
skin conditions such as
Psoriasis and Acne

Method of Use

Inhalation, Local Massage

Contra Indications

Can be skin irritant

Cajuput

The Cajuput tree is found in Australia, Malaysia and East India. The tree is a tall evergreen that can reach a height of 40ft (13.5m), it has thick pointed leaves and white flowers. The Cajuput tree is sometimes referred to as the 'crooked white tree' which is probably due to the fact that both the trunk and irregular branches have a white scaly bark which is easy to remove.

The leaves, twigs and buds are fermented before distillation.

The oil was used by the Malay and Indonesian peoples for its therapeutic properties long before its appearance in Europe in the mid 1600's.

In my opinion there are two reasons why the use of Cajuput should be left to the professional:
1. Cajuput can be a skin irritant
2. Cajuput is sometimes adulterated with other oils. The professional therapist can always check quality with his/her supplier.

The most common use I have for the oil is in a room burner or house spray when there is flu about. I have often used it this way to treat sinusitis.

As Cajuput is a powerful stimulant it should only be used in the evening if it is blended with a sedative oil such as Chamomile.

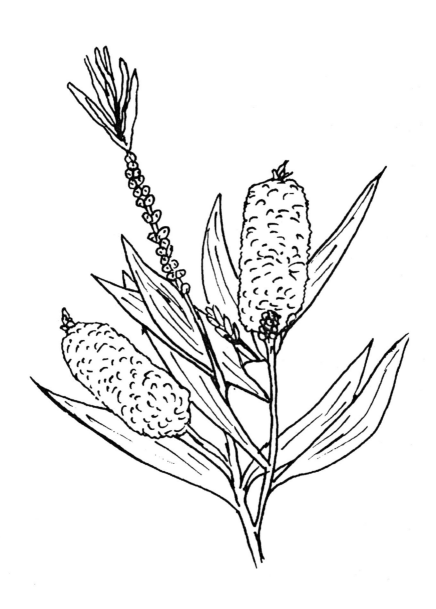

CAJUPUT

95

CHAMOMILE

Note	Middle
Botanical Name	Roman - Anthemis Nobilis German - Matricaria Chamomilla
Family	Compositae
Cultivation	Roman - Belgium, England, Morocco German - Hungary, Russia
Part of Plant	Flowers
Extracted by	Distillation
Yield 1 Gram Oil	Equals 100 grams base Material
Constituents	**Anthemis Nobilis:** **Sesquiterpene -** Azuline. **Acids -** Tiglic, Methacrylic, Angelic. **Matricaria Chamomilla:** **Sesquiterpene -** Azuline. **Aldehyde -** Cuminic.
Colour	Belgium/England - Pale blue, greenish blue to yellow

Colour	German - Deep blue (due to azulene)
Aroma	Sharp apple like
Blends Well With	Most oils, particularly Geranium, Lavender, Patchouli, Rose, Neroli, Ylang-Ylang, Jasmine, Marjoram
Properties	Analgesic, Antiallergenic, Anticonvulsive, Antidepressant, Antiemetic, Anti-inflammatory, Antiphlogistic, Antipruritic, Antirheumatic, Antiseptic, Diuretic, Emollient, Emmenagogue, Febrifuge, Hepatic, Nervine, Sedative, Splenetic, Stomachic, Sudorific, Tonic, Vermifuge, Vulnerary

Most Common Uses

Digestive   Diarrhoea, Flatulence,
                             Indigestion, Stomach ulcers

Gynaecological   Menstrual irregularity,
                             Menopausal symptoms

Neurological   Neuralgia

Emotional   Anxiety, Depression,
                             Insomnia

Skin   Acne, THread viens,
                             Mature, Dry, Burns

Other   Earache, Toothache

Like Lavender Chamomile is one of the most versatile oils

METHODS OF USE   Bath, Compress, Massage,
                        Inhalation, Vapourizer

CONTRA INDICATIONS   Pregnancy, Heavy periods

CHAMOMILE - ANTHEMIS NOBILIS

Cultivated mainly in Europe the plant grows up to 12 Inches (30 cm) high. It has a deep root and produces several stems some erect and some branched.

The leaves are pinnately divided into short and mainly hairy leafets. The flowers are arranged in terminal stemmed white ray flower heads, resembling the Daisy. Flowering time is mid Summer to early Autumn.

CHAMOMILE - MATRICARIA

A native of Europe and North West Africa this is an annual plant very similar to the Nobilis. The plant forms a clump with several erect smooth stems bearing finely divided hairless leaves and a solitary Daisy-like flower head. The flower head has an outer ray of white florets surrounding an inner yellow disk. The flower head of the Matricaria is much smaller than that of the nobilis.

GENERAL

The qualities and properties of both oils overlap. The Matricaria is much more blue and ink-like in colour.

Chamomile was considered sacred by the Egyptians and was used as a disinfectant in hospitals up to the Second World War. Some of the great herbalists of the past made claims for its uses which are still accepted today.

One of my favourite oils for complaints such as facial neuralgia, sinusitis, PMT, indigestion, earache. It is also a good oil to use for childhood problems such as sleeplessness, earache, tummy ache and diarrhoea.

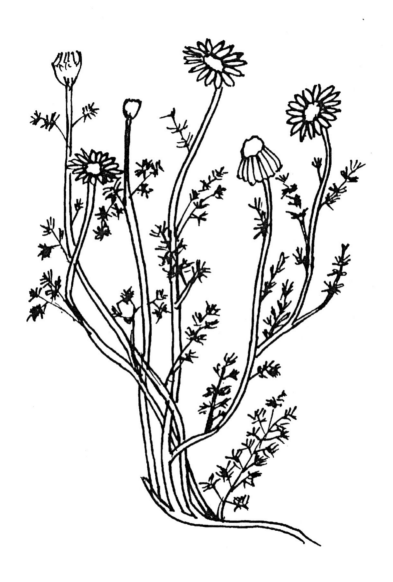

CHAMOMILE

101

CEDARWOOD

Note	Base
Botanical Name	Cedrus Atlantica & Juniperus Virginiana
Family	Cupresaceae/Coniferae
Cultivation	North Africa
Part of Plant	Wood
Extracted by	Distillation
Yield 1 Gram Oil	Equals 30 grams of base material
Constituents	**Sequiterpenes -** Cadinene, Cedrene, **Alcohol -** Cedrol, Cedrenol.
Colour	Yellow
Aroma	Woody/cedar
Blends Well With	Bergamot, Cypress, Jasmine, Neroli, Rosemary, Juniper, Lavender, Rose
Properties	Antiseptic, Astringent, Diuretic, Emollient, Expectorant, Fungicide, Insecticide, Sedative, Tonic

MOST COMMON USES

Respiratory	Infections, Catarrah, Coughs
Skin	Acne, Dandruff, Scalp disorders, Insect Repellent
Other	Urinary Infections, Cystitis, Vaginal Infections

METHOD OF USE

Bath, Massage, Inhalation

CONTRA INDICATIONS

Pregnancy
Sensitive skin

CEDARWOOD

If Jasmine and Rose are considered to be the King and Queen of the oils and flowers, surely the title of King of the trees and forests should be bestowed on this tall majestic evergreen that grows to about 100 ft (30 m) commanding space for its expansive branches.

The needles form in rosette bunches with barrel shaped upright cones and yellow flowers.

The Cedarwood can live for well over a thousand years. The wood is very aromatic and resists attack from insects; perhaps this is one reason why it was chosen by the Egyptians to build their ships, furniture and coffins (it was also used in mummification). The Temple of Solomon was built with Cedarwood. It is still used as a temple incense by the Tibetans. Today the red Cedarwood (Juniperous Virginiana) tends to be used for making smaller items such as pencils.

I use this oil for the following conditions:- In burners and sprays as an insect repellent. For chronic conditions such as arthritis/rheumatism and as a fixative for my perfumes.

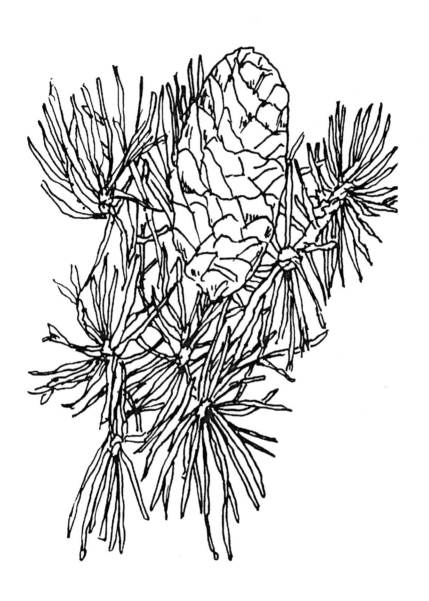

CEDARWOOD

CLARY SAGE

Note	Top/Middle
Botanical Name	Salvia Sclarea
Family	Labiatae
Cultivation	France, Russia, Morocco, Italy
Part of Plant	Flowering tops and foliage
Extracted by	Distillation
Yield 1 Gram Oil	Equals 800 grams base material
Constituents	**Sesquiterpene -** Caryophyllene. **Oxide-** Cineole. **Ester -** Linalyl acetate. **Alcohol -** Salviol, Linalool
Colour	Colourless, pale yellowish, greenish
Aroma	Sweet, Muscatel wine-like
Blends Well With	Cedarwood, Citrus, Geranium, Frankincense, Jasmine, Juniper, Lavender, Sandalwood

| Properties | Anticonvulsive, Antidepressant, Antiphlogistic, Antiseptic, Antispasmodic, Balsamic, Carminative, Deodorant, Digestive, Emmenagogue, Hypotensive, Nervine, Parturient, Sedative, Stomachic, Tonic, Uterine |

MOST COMMON USES

Emotional	Mental fatigue, Stress.
Respiratory	Asthma, Sore throats.
Circulatory	High blood pressure
Gynaecological	Menstrual problems, Infertility
Skin	Mature

| METHOD OF USE | Bath, Compress, Massage, Perfume, Vapouriser. |

| CONTRA INDICATIONS | Pregnancy; Before driving; Before or after the consumption of alcohol; May cause nightmares, sleepiness or skin irritation |

CLARY SAGE

A native to southern Europe though now cultivated world wide. Dry soil is important (damp soil rots the roots). The plant tends to hug the ground but can grow to 3 ft (90 cm). The leaves are large and grey-green in colour; they are heart shaped, wrinkled and pointed, and are covered with velvety hairs. The flowers are blue or white and bloom in August.

Clary Sage has many similar properties to Sage. One of its greater benefits is that it contains a far lower proportion of thujone, therefore does not present the risk of toxicity associated with Sage.

Both Sage and Clary Sage have a long history and were mentioned by Hippocrates, Dioscorides, Romans, Egyptians and the Herbals of the Middle Ages.

In Germany, Clary Sage was called Muscatel Sage and was used by some wine makers to enhance the flavour of cheap wines (makes them taste like true Muscatel). The results were, it is said, an exaggerated state of drunkenness.

Warning - Clary Sage should not be used on or by anybody who has consumed, or is about to consume, alcohol as this can cause drowsiness and in some cases severe nightmares.

Clary Sage is a very relaxing oil for the physical and emotional state; it should therefore be used with caution on people who are expected to have great mental clarity or to drive home after a treatment. For people who fall into these brackets the oil can be used either in the evening bath or a vapouriser.

Clary Sage is one of my favourite oils for the treatment of asthmathics and also for the treatment of abdominal cramp whether caused through digestive or menstrual problems.

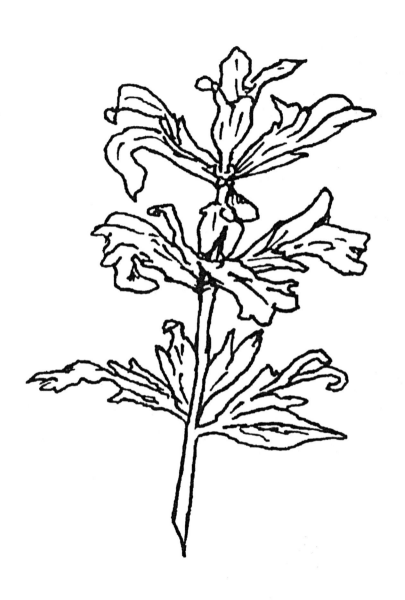

CLARY SAGE

CYPRESS

Note	Middle/Base
Botanical Name	Cupressus Sempervirens
Family	Coniferae/Cupresaceae
Cultivation	France, Germany
Part of Plant	Leaves/Cones
Extracted by	Distillation
Yield 1 Gram Oil	Equals 150 grams base material
Constituents	**Terpenes** - Camphene, Cymene, Pinene, Sylvestrene. **Ester** - Terpenyl acetate. **Aldehyde** - Furfural. **Alcohol** - Sabinol
Colour	Pale yellow
Aroma	Conifer
Blends Well With	Juniper, Lavender, Sandalwood, Clary-Sage, Rosemary, Bergamot, Lemon
Properties	Antirheumatic, Antiseptic, Antispasmodic, Astringent, Cicatrisant, Deodorant, Diuretic, Febrifuge, Haemostatic, Hepatic, Insecticide, Sedative, Styptic, Tonic, Vascoconstrictor

MOST COMMON USES

Emotional	Grief, Insomnia, Danger
Respiratory	Asthma, Coughing, Whooping Cough
Skin	Oily, Sweating, Palms, Feet
Digestive	Diarrhoea, Incontinence
Circulatory	Broken Veins, Fluid Retention, Varicose Veins, Haemorrhoids, Chilblains, Circulation, Cramp
Muscular	Tonic, Rheumatism, Cramp
Gynaecological	Painful Periods, Reduces abnormally heavy loss

METHOD OF USE

Bath, Compress, Massage, Vapourizer, Inhaler

CONTRA INDICATIONS

Pregnancy

CYPRESS

Family Cupressaceae sometimes known as the coniferous family. This name implies a particular needle-leaved tree due to the shape of their characteristic foliage. Another common family name is Conifer. This name implies the tree bears cones; a common feature of nearly all the group. The woody cones are made up of tough brown scales usually carrying two seeds. It is important for major suppliers to be aware of the true species being used for oil supply.

The Cypress is a tall vertical evergreen coniferous tree. It has been likened to a finger pointing to the heavens and can reach a height of up to 150 ft (45 m). The tree bears small flowers and brownish grey cones. The wood of the Cypress is reddish yellow, hard yet easy to work; this might be one reason why it was chosen by the Greeks for carving statues of their Gods and by the Phoenicians for building houses and ships.

The Greeks and Romans planted the tree in their cemeteries, possibly as a symbol for life after death, possibly because of its evergreen colour or indeed as its name "Sempervirens" suggests " lives forever".

The oil has many uses. I tend to favour it for the following : - asthmatic conditions, odema, heavy periods, varicose veins, piles, oily skin, and in particular sweaty feet.

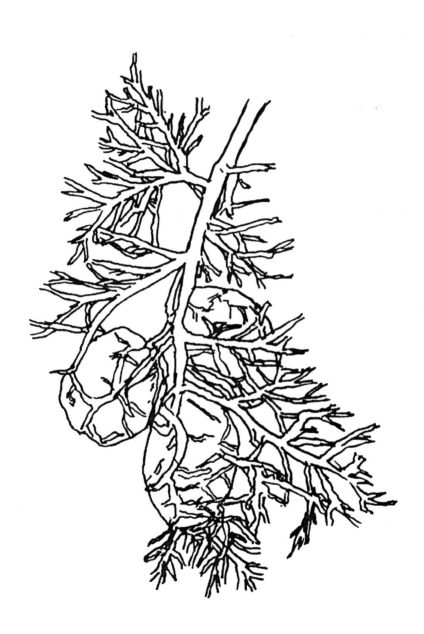

CYPRESS

EUCALYPTUS

Note	Top
Botanical Name	Eucalyptus Globulus
Family	Myrtaceae
Cultivation	Spain, Portugal, Australia, Tasmania, Zimbabwe
Part of Plant	Leaves
Extracted by	Distillation
Yield 1 Gram Oil	Equals 90 grams base material
Constituents	**Terpenes** - Camphene, Fenchene, Phellandrene, Pinene. **Oxide-** Cineole. **Aldehyde -** Citronellal
Colour	Pale yellow
Aroma	Eucalyptus
Blends Well With	Benzoin, Lavender, Juniper, Lemongrass, Melissa
Properties	Analgesic, Antirheumatic, Antiphlogistic, Antiseptic, Antispasmodic, Antiviral, Bactericide, Cicatrisant, Decongestant, Deodorant, Depurative, Diuretic, Expectorant, Febrifuge, Insecticide, Rubefacient, Stimulant, Vermifuge, Vulnerary

Most Common Uses

Emotional	Clears the mind, helps prevent drowsiness
Respiratory	Colds, Flu, Throat, Infections, Sinusitis, Asthma, Bronchitis, Dry cough
Skin	Boils, Pimples, Herpes simplex, Head lice
Muscular - Joints	Aches/Pains, Rheumatism, Arthritis
Other	Cystitis, Headaches

Methods of Use

Local Massage, Compress, Vaporizer, Local application to skin blemishes ie. Boils

Contra Indications

May irritate kidneys if used in high quantities. Can be a skin irritant. I do not recommend its use for facial massage. Protect face if oil is used in an inhaler. If using an a full body massage use at 1% to 1½% dilution

EUCALYPTUS

Nearly everyone can recognise this oil by its smell (it has a tendency to remind people of illness).

A native of Tasmania and Australia though now cultivated in European countries as well as California and North Africa. The common local name for Eucalyptus is the Gum Tree (due to the sweet smelling gum exuded by the bark). This oil was first distilled in Australia in the 1850's.

The eucalyptus tree is the tallest deciduous tree on our planet, growing to a height of over 450 ft (140-150m). The tree can reach 90 ft (27m) in just 20 years. The leaves of the young tree are round and a silvery bluish-green; where as those of the mature tree are long, pointed and yellowy-green. The oil gland are visible when the leaf is held up to the light. The flowers of the mature tree are a creamy white, the wood is very hard and the bark is smooth and pale grey in colour.

My favourite uses for this oil are :- Flu, Bronchitis, Fevers, Shingles and General Infections. I use it only in local massage never in a full body treatment.

I always use it in a spray or burner if a member of the household is suffering from any of these conditions. I also find it useful used in this manner when the usual childhood illnesses are in the family.

As an insect repellent in general Eucalyptus is excellent. Once a month I put a drop of blended oil on my dog's collar to keep him free from little visitors. Used in the same way the oil has a similar benefit for cats.

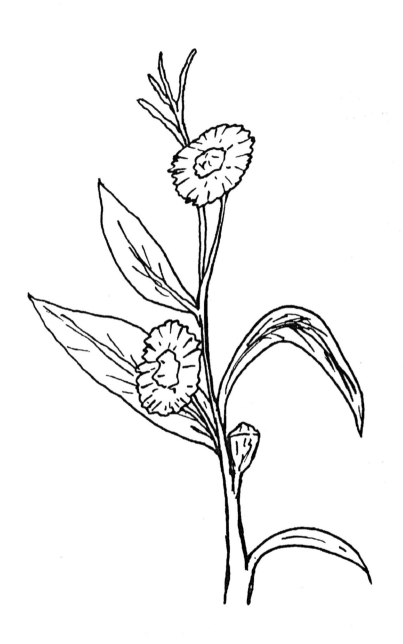

EUCALYPTUS

FENNEL SWEET

Note	Middle
Botanical Name	Foeniculum Vulgare
Family	Umbelliferae
Cultivation	India,America, Europe (Asia, Mediterranean)
Part of Plant	Seed
Extracted by	Distillation
Yield 1 Gram Oil	Equals 20 grams base material
Constituents	**Terpenes** - Camphene, Dipentene, Limonene, Phellandrene. **Phenols** - Anethole, Methylchavicol. **Ketone** - Fenchone. **Aldehydes** - Anisic, Cuminic
Colour	Colourless/pale yellow
Aroma	Warm/aniseed
Blends Well With	Geranium, Lavender, Rose, Sandalwood, Rosemary, Lemon
Properties	Antiphlogistic, Antiseptic, Antispasmodic, Detoxicant, Diuretic, Emmenagogue, Expectorant, Galactagogue

Most Common Uses

Digestive

Nausea, Flatulence,
Indigestion, Colic,
Hiccoughs, Colitis

Gynaecological

Scanty, Painful periods,
PMS.

Other

Cellulite, Urine Retention,
Urinary Tract Infection
Mouth Wash

Methods of Use

Bath, Compress, Massage
Mouth Wash

Contra Indications

Children
Pregnancy
Epilepsy
Can be a skin irritant
Diabetic

FENNEL

The plant is a native of the Mediterranean area though it is now cultivated in many parts of the globe. It can grow to about 5 - 6 feet (1.5 - 2 metres) high with feathery blue green leaves and large umbells of yellow flowers about 6 inches (15 cms) across, appearing from July to October, followed by greenish yellow or brownish seeds.

The history of fennel goes back a long way; it was known to the Chinese, Indians, Egyptians, Greeks and Romans. Theophrastus, Pliney, Dioscorides and Hippocrates all mentioned its benefits. The Roman soldiers are said to have carried the seeds on long treks to chew when they were hungry.

Fennel is considered a useful oil for the female reproductive system. Its effects have been known for centuries. It is now thought that this could be due to a hormone, a form of oestrogen, in its structure.

My own main uses for the oil are for all digestive problems; PMS; scant periods; painful periods; cellulite and fluid retention.

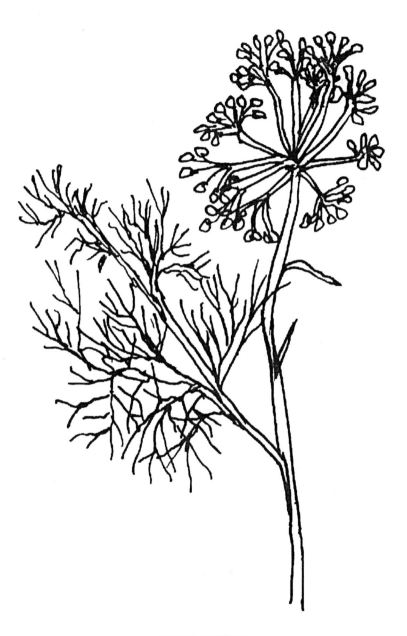

FENNEL

FRANKINCENSE

Note	Middle/Base
Botanical Name	Boswellia Thurifera
Family	Burseraceae
Cultivation	North Africa
Part of Plant	Resin
Extracted by	Distillation
Yield 1 Gram Oil	Equals 12 grams base material
Constituents	**Terpenes** - Camphene, Dipentene, Pinene, Phellandrene. **Sesquiterpene** - Cadinene. **Alcohol** - Olibanol
Colour	Colourless / pale yellow yellowish brown
Aroma	Camphorous/Penetrating with a slight hint of lemon
Blends Well With	Basil, Black Pepper, Citrus oils, Geranium, Lavender, Sandalwood, Melissa
Properties	Antiseptic, Astringent, Digestive, Diuretic, Sedative

Most Common Uses

Skin

Stretch marks, Mature,
Slack, Wrinkled,
Inflammation, Boils,
Pimples

Respiratory

Pulmonary Antiseptic,
Coughs/colds, Bronchial
Catarrh, Asthma

Emotional

Anxiety

Gynaecological

Heavy periods

Other

Uterine tonic, Gout

Methods of Use

Massage, Face creams,
Lotions, Local application
on skin blemishes

Contra Indications

This seems to be a safe oil
but like all essential oils
needs to be used with care

FRANKINCENSE

Also known as Olibanum, is a native of the Middle East and Africa. The small tree has abundant pinnate leaves and white to pale pink flowers.

The highly aromatic resin permeates the leaves and bark of the tree and even exudes as a milky juice from the flowers. It is reported that the bedouins of the past used to visit all the trees in succession and make a deep incision in each; peeling off a narrow strip of bark just below the wound. For the next three months this exercise would be repeated at monthly intervals; each time the original incision would be made deeper.

The large tears are whitish yellow and waxy. They tend to solidify into a yellowish amber colour varying in size from a pea to a walnut. These would be scraped off into large baskets. Every two weeks the harvesters would return to collect the resin until the first rains came and put a close on the year's gatherings.

Frankincense was amongst the most costly substance in the ancient world. It has been used since ancient time in religious rituals and is still used today in incense burners. It was one of the gifts brought to Jesus by the three wise men.

I use the oil in the main for the following conditions:-
Asthmathics, bronchitis, coughing, heavy periods, mature skin care, anxiety.

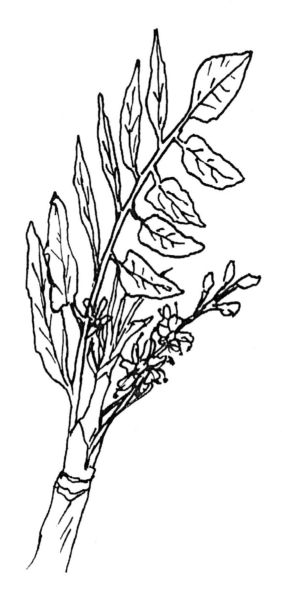

FRANKINCENSE

GERANIUM

Note	Middle
Botanical Name	Pelargonium Graveolens Pelargonium Odorantissimum
Family	Geraniaceae
Cultivation	France, Spain, Italy, Morocco, Egypt (Native Africa)
Part of Plant	Leaves/Flowers
Extracted by	Steam Distillation
Yield 1 Gram Oil	Equals 40 grams base material
Constituents	**Terpene** - Sabinene. **Phenol** - Eugenol. **Ketone** - Menthone. **Aldehyde** - Citral. **Alcohols** - Geraniol, Citronellol, Linalool, Myrtenol, Terpineol. **Acid** - Geranic
Colour	Greenish Yellow

Aroma	Rich Sweet Rose Like, Graveolens, Slight apple-like = Odorantissimum
Blends Well With	Most oils but especially Basil, Lavender, All Citrus, Rose, Jasmine, Neroli, Petitgrain
Properties	Analgesic, Antidepressant, Antiseptic, Astringent, Cicatrisant, Cytophylactic, Diuretic, Deodorant, Haemostatic, Insecticide, Styptic, Tonic, Vasoconstrictor

Most Common Uses

Respiratory System	Colds, Flu, Throat, Mouth Infections
Skin	Acne, Dry Eczema, Herpes Simplex, Stretchmarks, Soothes measles and general rashes
Head	Dandruff, Head lice
Digestive	Diarrhoea, Gastroenteritis
Gynaecological	Hormone inbalance, PMS, Menopausal
Other	Fluid Retention, Cellulite, Urinary Tract Infections, Diabetes

Method of Use

Bath, Compress, Massage, Vaporizer, Perfume

CONTRA INDICATIONS

Pregnancy
Insomniacs especially at
night time
Can cause allergic reactions

GERANIUM

Pelargonium Graveolens is a perennial plant which grows to about 2 - 3 ft (1 m). It has pointed serrated edged leaves and small pink flowers. Although a native of Africa the plant is cultivated in a number of countries. Many species of Pelargonium exist, but only about five are used in the production of essential oil. These include Pelargonium Graveolens; Pelargonium Odoratissimum; Pelargonium Capitatum; Pelargonium Roseum (Rose Geranium) and Pelargonium Radula.

Geranium oil is often used to adulterate Rose oil. Geranium itself is quite expensive, so once again, be warned that there are no bargains in essential oil of quality. The most expensive oil comes from the Reunion, an island in the South West Indian ocean.

The 19th century saw the first distillation of essential oils from France. There is not a lot of information about geranium in the history books until Culpepper's Herbal was published in 1653; although mention had previously been made by Dioscorides about a "Geranion". However, we are unsure if this was reference to the same plant (Geranium).

Geranium is an adrenal cortex stimulant.
I find Geranium to be a most useful oil and use it for the following conditions:
Menopausal symptoms; PMS.; fluid retention; cellulite; depression; all skin types (as a balancer); insect repellent and air freshener/deodoriser.

130

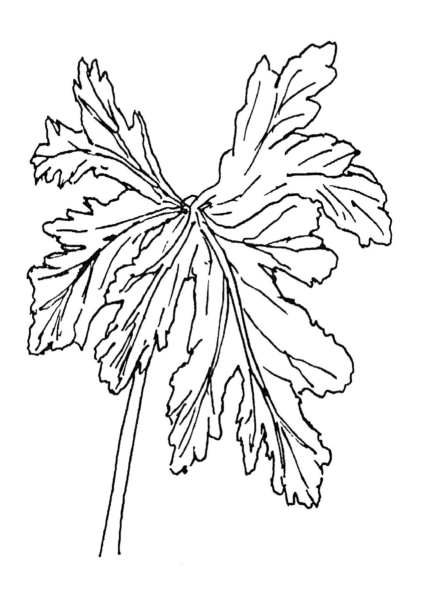

GERANIUM

GINGER

Note	Base
Botanical Name	Zingiber Officinale
Family	Zingiberaceae
Cultivation	India, China
Part of Plant	Roots
Extracted by	Distillation
Yield 1 Gram Oil	Equals 40 grams base material
Constituents	**Terpenes** - Camphene, Limonene, Phellandrene. **Sesquiterpene** - Zingiberene. **Oxide** - Cineole. **Aldehyde** - Citral. **Alcohol** - Borneol
Colour	Pale greenish yellow, deep yellow
Aroma	Fresh root ginger/sweet/ woody
Blends Well With	Citrus, Eucalyptus, Frankinscence, Geranium, Rosemary
Properties	Analagesic, Antiemetic, Antiseptic, Antiscorbutic, Aperitif, Aphrodisiac, Carminative, Expectorant, Febrifuge, Laxative, Rubefacient, Stimulant, Stomachic, Sudorific, Tonic

Most Common Uses

Muscular - Joints	Rheumatic pain, Muscular pain, Arthritis
Respiratory	Catarrh, Colds, Flu, Sore Throats
Digestive	Diarrhoea, Travel sickness
Other	Room Burner for morning sickness of pregnancy

Methods of Use	Compress, Local massage, Vaporizer

Contra Indication	Can be a Skin Irritant (use in low dilutions) Do not use prior to exposure to U.V. Sun/ Sunbed

GINGER

A perennial plant with reed-like leaves and thick rhizomes which are tube-like and knotted on both sides.

Ginger was mentioned in old Chinese manuscripts. It was also known to the Greeks and Romans, but was not discovered in Europe until the middle ages.

Ginger contains about 2% volatile oil. It is sensitive to strong sunlight and so is grown in the shade of other crops.

When the stems dry off the tubers are ready for harvesting.

The most common use I have for this oil is for treating localised areas of muscular type pain.

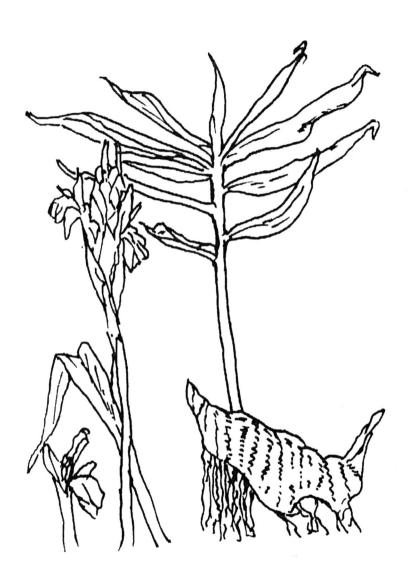

GINGER

GRAPEFRUIT

Note	Top
Botanical Name	Citrus Paradisi
Family	Rutaceae
Cultivation	USA
Part of Plant	Rind of fruit
Extracted by	Expression
Yield 1 Gram Oil	Equals 250 grams base material
Constituents	**Terpenes** - Limonene, Pinene. **Aldehyde** - Citral. **Alcohols** - Geraniol, Linalool
Colour	Yellow/greenish
Aroma	Tangy
Blends Well With	Most other oils
Properties	Antidepressant, Digestive, Stimulant, Tonic

Most Common Uses

Emotional	Mental stimulant
Digestive	Indigestion, Liver and Gallbladder problems

Contra Indications

Young children
Exposure to Ultra Violet
Sun/Sunbed

GRAPEFRUIT

The Grapefruit grows on a fairly tall sturdy tree approximately 18 ft (6 m) tall with dense foliage of dark green, glossy leaves. The large white flowers are borne single or in clusters in the axils of the leaves. Mature trees produce large crops of the fruit (up to 1500 lbs per tree).

The fruit which is yellow when ripe, ranges from 4-6 inches (100 -150 mm) in diameter, twice the size of the average orange. It became a well established fruit in the islands of the West Indies before coming to the mainland USA. Other producing countries include Israel, Brazil and South Africa.

The essential oil is best when expressed. A slightly inferior oil is distilled.

I tend to reach for the grapefruit oil most often when treating people with stress related problems. I find also that the Grapefruit added to a floral oil helps to give the aroma a more sharp but pleasing smell.

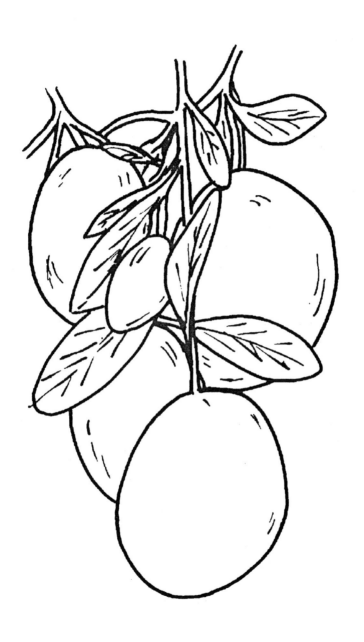

GRAPEFRUIT

139

JASMINE

Note	Middle/Base
Botanical Name	Jasminum Officinale or Jasminum Grandiflorum
Family	Oleaceae/Jasminaceae
Cultivation	France, Algeria, Egypt, Morocco, China
Part of Plant	Flowers
Extracted by	Enfleurage, Solvent extraction
Yield 1 Gram Oil	Equals 900 grams base material
Constituents	**Phenol** - Eugenol. **Ketone** - Jasmone. **Esters** - Linalyl acetate, Methyl anthranilate. **Alcohols** - Benzyl, Farnesol, Geraniol, Nerol, Terpineol
Colour	Reddish brown
Aroma	Floral, sweet, slightly heady
Blends Well With	All oils but especially citrus

Properties	Antidepressant, Antiseptic, Antispasmodic, Aphrodisiac, Emollient, Galactagogue, Parturient, Sedative, Uterine

MOST COMMON USES

Emotional	Depression, Tension, Anxiety, Confidence
Gynaecological	Menstrual pain/cramp, Labour pains
Other	Male prostate gland, Dry skin, Dry coughs

METHODS OF USE	Bath, Compress, Massage, Vapouriser, Perfume

CONTRA INDICATION	Pregnancy - (may be used at point of labour) Overuse may have opposite to desired effect Caution - use in low dilutions

141

JASMINE

The common name of Jasmine is used for the genus Jasminum of the Oleaceae family (Olive family). Personally I prefer this fragrance to all others.

A vine-like deciduous shrub which grows to over 30 ft high. It has long smooth, slender branches with oval pointed leaves. The pin-wheel shaped white flower head grows on a thin pedicel and opens at night. This night opening is the reason the flowers have to be picked at night. At this time the odour is at its most powerful.

The plant originates from Iran and India though it is now grown in Egypt, Morocco, Italy and France. France is now a major producer.

Jasmine is one of the most expensive oils to purchase, however only a very small amount is necessary, as low as 1 drop in 10 or even 20 ml of base.

Jasmine is classified amongst the aphrodisiacs and is important to the perfumery industry as no synthetic equivalent has been created. The oil is used in Femme by Rochas, Chanel No 5 and Samsara by Guerlain. Some perfume houses have resorted to buying their own Jasmine fields.

I use it mainly for the following conditions :- Scant periods, PMS., nervousness, lack of self esteem, frigidity.

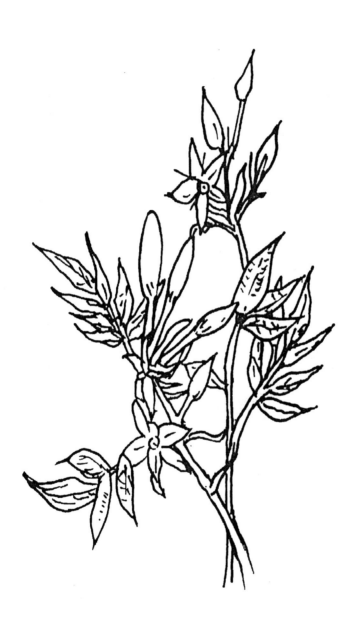

JASMINE

JUNIPER

Note	Middle
Botanical Name	Juniperus Communis
Family	Cupressaceae/Coniferae
Cultivation	Yugoslavia, Italy, France
Part of Plant	Ripe Berries
Extracted by	Distillation
Yield 1 Gram Oil	Equals 100 grams base material
Constituents	**Terpenes** - Camphene, Myrcene, Pinene, Sabinene. **Sesquiterpenes** - Cadinene, Cedrene. **Alcohols** - Borneol, Terpineol
Colour	Colourless/pale greenish-yellow
Aroma	Slight turpentine, Balsmic, Hot, Woody
Blends Well With	Rosemary, Cypress, Lavender, Sandalwood, Geranium, Bergamot, Frankincense

Properties	Antiseptic, Antirheumatic, Antispasmodic, Aphrodisiac, Astringent, Carminative, Cicatrisant, Depurative, Detoxicant, Diuretic, Emmenagogue, Nervine, Insecticide, Parturient, Rubefacient, Stimulating Stomachic, Sudorific, Tonic, Vulnerary

MOST COMMON USES

Muscular	Aches, Pain, Rheumatism
Digestive	Indigestion, Flatulence, Diarrhoea, Colic
Emotional	Anxiety/Stress
Skin	Acne, Oily, Congested, Seborrhoea of scalp
Other	Scanty Periods, Fluid Retention

METHODS OF USE

Bath, Massage, Vaporiser

CONTRA INDICATIONS

Do not use in Pregnancy

JUNIPER

An evergreen shrub found in dry soil it usually grows to a height of 12 ft (2 - 4m) though has been known to grow as tall as 25 ft (7m). The bark is a dark brown tinged with red. A pretty coloured shrub, Juniper's needle-shaped leaves have white stripes on top and shiny yellow/green underneath. On the male tree the flowers are yellow.

Flowering time is April to June. The berry fruit is green in the first year ripening to a blue black with a grey tinge in the second.

Reference to Juniper was made by the Egyptians and Greeks. The Romans used it as an antiseptic; Galean and Pliny mentioned its use for liver complaints and St. Hildegarde prescribed it for pulmonary infections.

Herbalists throughout the ages have mentioned the virtues of Juniper. I have used the oil in a wash for dogs with fleas and after blending in vodka and distilled water, have sprayed it on cats.

For humans I find this oil most useful when treating congested spotty skin on the back (blended with Tea-Tree).

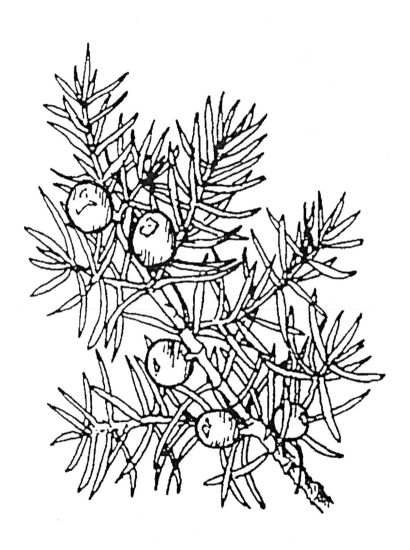

JUNIPER

147

LAVENDER

Middle/Base

Lavendula Officinalis
Lavendula Angustifolia

Family	Labiatae
Cultivation	France, England, Spain, USSR
Part of Plant	Flowers
Extracted by	Distillation
Yield 1 Gram Oil	Equals 145 grams base material
Constituents	**Terpenes** - Limonene, Pinene. **Sesquiterpene** - Caryophyllene. **Oxide** - Cineole. **Ester** - Geranyl acetate, Lavandulyl acetate, Linalyl acetate. **Alcohols** - Borneol, Geraniol, Lavandulol, Linalool.
Colour	Pale Yellow, yellowish-green
Aroma	Classical, mossy/woody
Blends Well With	Most oils, Citrus, Clary-sage, Bergamot, Geranium, Patchouli, Rosemary; though less well with the exotic such as Ylang-Ylang, Jasmine, etc.

Properties	Analgesic, Anticonvulsive, Antidepressant, Antiphlogistic,Antirheumatic, Antiseptic Antispasmodic, Antiviral, Bactericide, Bechic Carminative, Cholagogue, Cicatrisant, Cordial, Cytophylactic,Decongestant, Deodorant, Detoxicant, Diuretic, Emmenagogue, Fungicidal, Hypnotic, Hypotensive, Immuno-stimulant, Nervine, Restorative, Sedative, Splenetic, Sudorific, Tonic, Vulnerary
MOST COMMON USES	Burns, Bites, Stings, Insomnia, Anxiety, Nervous Tension, Immune Deficiency, Lice, Eczema/ Dermatitis
METHODS OF USE	Bath, Compress, Massage, Inhaler, Vapouriser
CONTRA INDICATIONS	Pregnancy. Use with caution - Asthma, Hayfever Blood Pressure. Over use might overstimulate

LAVENDER

A fragrant spreading shrub with grey green narrow, linear downy leaves and purple-blue flowers that are borne on long slender stems. The plant reaches a height of about 3 ft (1m).

The Lavender originates from the Mediterranean though it is now cultivated in most parts of the world including Norfolk U.K. Lavender from the famous Grasse area of France is prized for its strong sweet fragrance. The English Lavender has a slightly more camphoric smell. In the 1700's the lavender fields of Mitcham, Surrey were harvested by the perfumers Yardley.

Before the invention of modern machinery the farmers of old would climb the mountains in the scorching mid day sun to cut the Lavender, tie it into bundles and carry it on their backs down the mountainside to the village still, where all the varieties of Lavender were distilled together. Today this work is done mainly by machines harvesting the lavender from Lavender fields; with the Lavenders being classified and distilled separately.

The whole plant is highly aromatic. The best quality oil is produced from the flowers though some oil is produced from the stalk and the leaves.

Lavender like a lot of our aromatherapy oils has a long history, being mentioned by Dioscorides, Galen, Pliny and St. Hildegrade. The Romans used it in their wounds and added it to their bath water. It was popular in The Elizabethan, Stuart and even Victorian times; Lavender sachets were sewn into dress and skirt hems and placed in linen cupboards. Dr Jean Valnet , an army surgeon, used the oils to treat the war wounded. In more modern times Lavender was made famous by the French chemist Dr René Gattefosse when he severely burned his hand in the laboratory and plunged it into the nearest bowl of liquid; it transpired that the bowl contained Lavender oil. The pain eased and the burn healed very quickly. It is Dr René Gattefosse who coined the word Aromathérapie.

Every household should have a bottle of Lavender in the First Aid Box. It is the most versatile and most commonly used of all oils with an odour that is second in popularity only to that of Rose or Jasmine and it blends well with almost all other oils.

I use Lavender in the main to treat the following conditions:- acne, burns, bites, stings, bruises, cuts, grazes, cystitis, leucorrhoea, rheumatic conditions, gout, colds, flu, cold sores, shingles, insect repellant, insomnia, migraine, childhood illnesses (very low dilutions, as little as ¼% up to 1% depending on age).

All childhood illnesses should be medically investigated.

Lavender is one of the few oils that can be applied neat to the skin. **If treating a burn use neat oil,** not blended, then cover the area with a cold damp gauze or hankie (not cotton wool). Normal treatment for a burn is to plunge the burn into ice cold water or put under a cold running tap until pain eases. If Lavender oil is available use next.

Serious burns need medical attention.

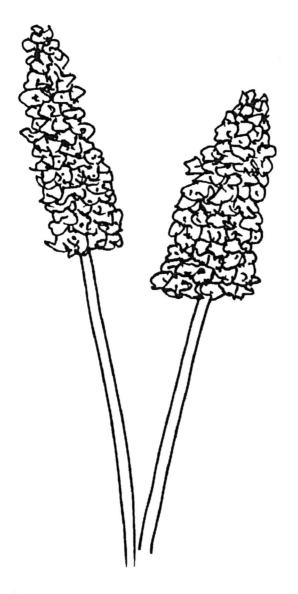

LAVENDER

LEMON

Note	Top
Botanical Name	Citrus Limonum
Family	Rutaceae
Cultivation	India, Italy, Spain, California (Mediterranean)
Part of Plant	Fruit peel
Extracted by	Expression
Yield 1 Gram Oil	Equals 200 grams base material
Constituents	**Terpenes -**, Camphene, Dipentene, Limonene, Pinene, Phellandrene. **Sesquiterpenes -** Bisabolene, Cadinene. **Aldehydes -** Citral, Citronellal. **Alcohol -** Linalool
Colour	Pale Yellow/yellowish green
Aroma	Lemon
Blends Well With	Lavender, Neroli, and all the floral and exotic oils
Properties	Antiscorbutic, Antineuralgic, Antirheumatic, Antipruritic, Antiseptic, Astringent, Bactericide, Carminative, Cicatrisant,

	Diuretic, Emollient, Febrifuge, Haemostatic, Hepatic, Insecticide, Laxative, Tonic
MOST COMMON USES	
Respiratory	Throat Infections, Colds, Flu
Skin	Greasy, Herpes Simplex, Cuts, Wounds, Boils, Spots, Brightens dull discoloured skins
Muscular - Joints	Arthritis, Rheumatism
Digestive	Heartburn, Gastric Acidity, Indigestion, Liver
Circulation	High Blood Pressure, Varicose Veins, Sluggish Circulation
Other	Cellulite, Fluid Retention, Haemorrhoids, Kidney Diabetic. Household antiseptic Mouth Wash
METHODS OF USE	Compress, Local Massage, Vapouriser
CONTRA INDICATIONS	Exposure to Ultra Violet. Can be a skin irritant

LEMON

The Lemon is a small thorny evergreen that grows up to about 16 ft (5m).

The Lemon Tree originates in China, India and Japan but is now cultivated in the USA and in many Mediterranean countries especially Italy, Spain, France, Sicily and Cyprus.

The leaves of the Lemon tree are egg-shaped and slightly scalloped. The white flowers appear singularly or in pairs. The fruit of this tree is too well known to warrant description.

The oil was used in French hospitals as a disinfectant up to the First World War. Most people like the fragrance of Lemon oil.

I find I use this oil most for the treatment of:- Sweaty feet, air disinfectant, varicose veins, insect bites, bronchitis, laryngitis, hand treatments.

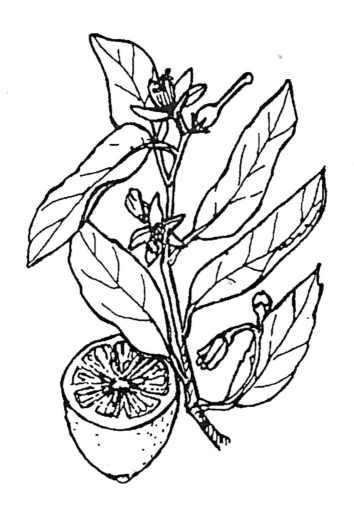

LEMON

157

LEMONGRASS

Note	Top
Botanical Name	Cymbopogan Citratus
Family	Gramineae
Cultivation	Brazil, Central Africa, Malay, Madras
Part of Plant	Leaves
Extracted by	Distillation
Yield 1 Gram Oil	Equals 15 grams base material
Constituents	**Terpenes** - Limonene, Myrcene. **Aldehydes** - Citral, Citronellal. **Alcohols** - Farnesol, Geraniol, Nerol
Colour	Yellow/golden, reddish/brown
Aroma	Fresh lemony
Blends Well With	Geranium, Jasmine, Lavender, Rosemary, Rose, Neroli, Tea-Tree
Properties	Antidepressant, Antiseptic, Bacteriacide, Carminative, Deodorant, Diuretic, Fungicide, Insecticide, Stimulant, Tonic

MOST COMMON USES	Feverish Conditions, Infectious diseases, Gastroenteritis, Colitis, Fungal Infections
Other	Insect repellant, Household Antiseptic
METHODS OF USE	Local massage, Foot bath, Vapouriser
CONTRA INDICATIONS	Can be a skin irritant, use in low dilution

LEMONGRASS

A fragrant tropical grass which grows up to 3 ft (1m) high. It reproduces by root division.

A native of Asia now cultivated in India, Sri Lanka, Indonesia, Africa as well as North and South America. The Lemongrass is a member of the family of tropical grasses like Palmarosa-Vetiver and Citronella.

Between two and three crops of grass are cut each year. This tends to exhaust a soil that is not properly fertilised and means that the grasses have to be moved to new ground every few years in order to sustain the quality.

I personally use this oil for tired aching muscles especially after long journeys sitting down. I use it also as an insect repellant spray or in a room burner to liven up my party guests.

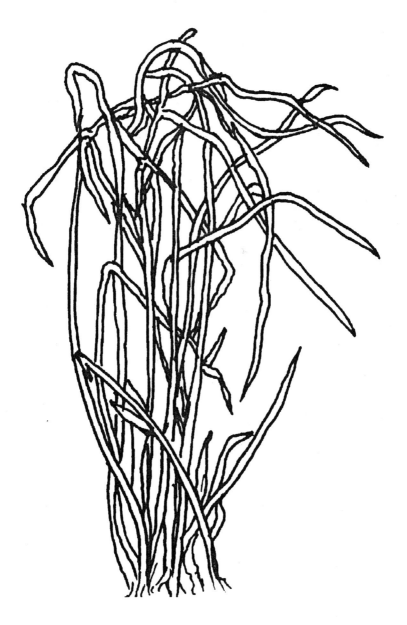

LEMONGRASS

MANDARIN

Note	Top
Botanical Name	Citrus Madurensis
Family	Rutaceae
Cultivation	Brazil,Spain,Italy, California.
Part of Plant	Peel
Extracted by	Expression
Yield 1 Gram Oil	Equals 150 grams of base material
Constituents	**Terpene** - Limonene. **Ester** - Methyl Anthranilate. **Aldehydes** - Citral Citronellal. **Alcohol** - Geraniol
Colour	Golden with a faint blue tint which becomes visible in bright light.
Aroma	Delicate, sweet, tangy with floral undertones.
Blends Well With	Most oils, Bergamot, Lavender, Marjoram, Black Pepper, Neroli, Chamomile, Rose.

Properties	Antispasmodic, Emollient, Cholagogue, Cytophylactic, Digestive, Sedative, Tonic

MOST COMMON USES

Depression, Anxiety,
Stress Flatulence,
Irritability
PMS, Stimulates Appetite,
Stimulates Liver, Stretch
Marks, Scarring,

Other

Insomnia
Rich in vitamin C
Perfume

METHODS OF USE

Bath, Compress, Massage,
Vapouriser

CONTRA INDICATIONS

Do not use prior to
exposure to ultra violet light
(sun or sunbed).
Overdose can have a
hypnotic effect

MANDARIN

A native of China and the Far East, Mandarin was brought to
Europe at the beginning of the 19th century. It is an evergreen
with small glossy leaves and fragrant flowers. The tree grows
to about 20 ft (6 m) in height and bears a very sweet yellowy
fruit which contains pips.

My main use for Mandarin is to blend with the heavy floral
oils to give a more pleasing smell and also to treat general
digestive and liver problems. I will, on occasion, use this oil
to treat skin recovering from acne.

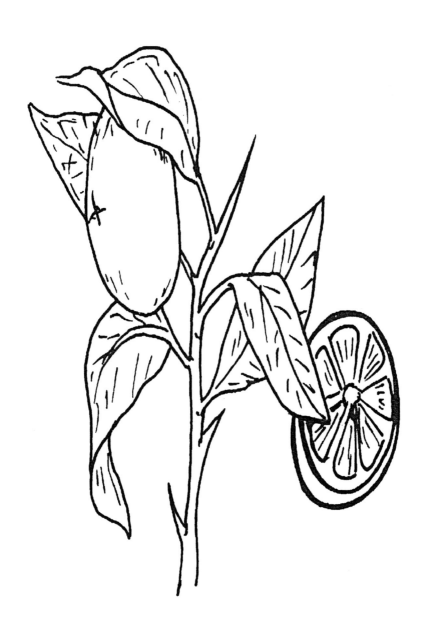

MANDARIN

165

MARJORAM

Note	Middle
Botanical Name	Origanum Marjorana
Family	Labiatae
Cultivation	Spain, France, Tunisia
Part of Plant	Flowering tops/leaves
Extracted by	Distillation
Yield 1 Gram Oil	Equals 200 grams base material
Constituents	**Terpenes** - Pinene, Sabinene, Terpinene. **Sesquiterpene** - Caryophyllene. **Ketone** - Camphor. **Alcohols** - Borneol, Terpineol.
Colour	Yellowish/dark brown
Aroma	Spicy, slightly peppery
Blends Well With	Bergamot, Lemon, Lavender, Rosemary, Rosewood, Ylang-Ylang
Properties	Analgesic, Anaphrodisiac, Antiseptic, Antispasmodic, Carminative, Cephalic, Cordial, Digestive, Emmenagogue, Expectorant, Hypotensive, Laxative, Nervine, Sedative, Tonic, Vulnerary

Most Common Uses

Emotional	Anxiety, Tension, Hysteria, Loneliness, Grief, Insomnia
Respiratory	Asthma, Colds, Bronchitis
Vascular	High Blood Pressure (dilates arteries)
Muscular	Cramps, Aches/Pains, Sprains/Strains, Rheumatism, Arthritis
Neurological	Neuralgia
Digestive	Colic, Constipation, Indigestion, Flatulence
Gynaecological	Menstrual Cramp, Period Pain

Methods of Use

Bath Compress, Massage, Vapouriser, Inhaler

Contra Indications

Pregnancy
Alcohol
Low Blood Pressure
Can cause drowsiness -
Beware if the
recipient is to use any
mechanical or electrical
equipment after treatment.
Can have a stupefying
effect if not used with care

MARJORAM

The plant known as sweet or knotted Marjoram is a small shrub which can grow to a height of about 20 inches (50 cm). It is native to the Mediterranean region although it is cultivated widely.

The stems, red to brownish red, are mainly upright and stout. The flowers are small white or pink in colour and arranged in small rounded spikes. Flowering time is mid-summer to early Autumn.

St. Hildegarde thought it a cure for leprosy. Dioscorides recommended it for animal bites, the Romans used it to drive away ants and the Greeks used it to treat spasm (Theophrastus mentioned it as a medicinal plant). During the middle ages it was used not only in a medicinal role but also in superstition. Nearer to present time, in the 1600's, nosegays contained Marjoram to mask unpleasant smells.

My uses for this oil are many, but in particular for :-
high blood pressure, heart conditions, asthma, menstrual cramp, intestinal cramp, rheumatism/arthritis, insomnia, and on aching/painful muscles after exercise.

The oil has a strong smell which is acceptable to both males and females and is considered an anti-aphrodisiac. This is brought about not by hormonal reaction but by the oil's lessening effects on the emotional level.

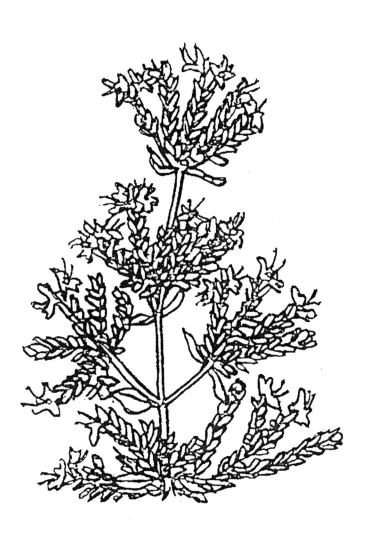

MARJORAM

MELISSA

Note	Middle
Botanical Name	Melissa Officinalis
Family	Labiatae
Cultivation	France some USA, (Mediterranean)
Part of Plant	Leaves/Flowers
Extracted by	Distillation
Yield 1 Gram Oil	Equals 900 grams base material
Constituents	**Sesquiterpene** - Caryophyllene. **Ester** - Geranyl acetate. **Aldehydes** - Citral, Citronellal. **Alcohols** - Citronellol, Geraniol, Linalool. **Acid** - Citronellic
Colour	Very pale brownish
Aroma	Fresh lemony
Blends Well With	Geranium, Lavender, Neroli, Ylang-Ylang, Jasmine, Rose, Rosemary, Chamomile

Properties	Antiallergenic, Antidepressant, Antispasmodic, Carminative, Cordial, Digestive, Febrifuge, Hypotensive, Nervine, Sedative, Stomachic, Tonic, Uterine

MOST COMMON USES

Emotional	Depression, Insomnia, Migraine, Anxiety, Emotional Shock, Grief, Shingles, Cold Sores
Other	Flatulence High blood pressure

METHODS OF USE	Bath, Compress, Massage, Vapouriser

CONTRA INDICATIONS	Can be a skin irritant use in low dilutions

Important Note:- Melissa is sometimes called Citronelle or Lemon Balm. Melissa is a very expensive oil, produced in very small quantities, very often adulterated especially with Lemongrass and/or Citronella (Cymbopogon-Nardus) of the Family Graminae

MELISSA

A native of Southern Europe, this strong perennial has small green slightly hairy, wrinkled leaves and tiny yellowish white flowers and grows to about 2 feet (60 cms) tall. During May and June the plant is harvested prior to the flower opening. The name derives from the latin name for honey. Bees seem to love the Melissa plant. Theophrastuc and Dioscorides wrote about the "bee plant". In the 14th century a group of French Carmelite nuns produced a tonic water containing Melissa.

I use the oil most often when treating the following conditions: shock; bereavement; asthma; high blood pressure or irregular periods.

I would suggest that this oil is used only by the more experienced therapist who is absolutely sure of the origin and purity of the oil.

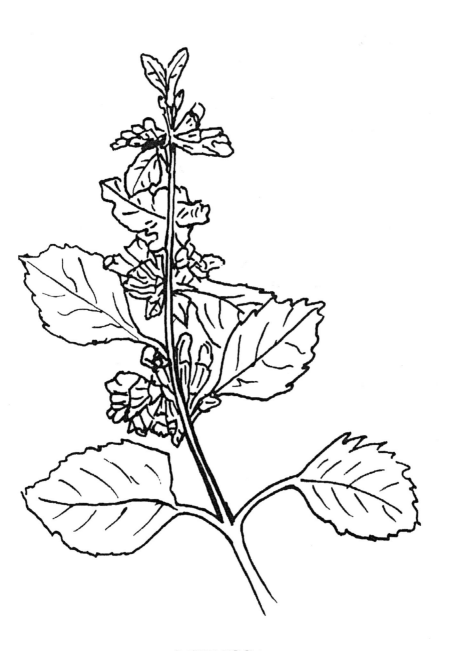

MELISSA

MYRRH

Note	Base
Botanical Name	Commiphora myrrha
Family	Burseraceae
Cultivation	North Eastern Africa, Libya
Part of Plant	Resin from trunk
Extracted by	Steam Distillation
Yield 1 Gram Oil	Equals 15 grams base material
Constituents	**Terpenes** - Dipentene, Limonene, Heerabolene, Pinene. **Sesquiterpenes** - Cadinene. **Phenols** - Eugenol. **Aldehydes** - Cinnamic, Cuminic. **Acids** -Myrrholic
Colour	Pale yellow
Aroma	Musty, incense-like
Blends Well With	Camphor, Lavender
Properties	Antiseptic, Astringent, Anti-inflammatery, Emmenagogue Expectorant,Fungicidal, Sedative, Tonic, Uterine, Vulnerary

MOST COMMON USES

Skin
Slow healing wounds,
Eczema, Athlete's foot,
Chapped skin, Mouth
ulcers, Gum disorders

Respiratory
Chest infections, Catarrh,
Chronic Bronchitis, Colds,
Sore throats

Digestive
Diarrhoea, Flatulence,
Tonic

Other
Thrush, Haemorrhoids,
Loss of appetite

CONTRA INDICATIONS
Pregnancy

MYRRH

A good sized bushy tree growing to about 9 ft (3 m). The trifoliate leaves are scanty and aromatic growing on sturdy knotted branches. The flowers are small and white.

Myrrh was first recognised in the early 19th century in a place known as Ghizan on the Red Sea coast, an area so dry and barren that it is called Tehama meaning "Hell".

The Myrrh bush has natural ducts in the bark. The tissue between the ducts breaks down forming cavities. These cavities become filled with a granular secretion. When, either through natural fissures or through incision the bark is broken, a thick pale yellow liquid flows out. This liquid hardens to a reddish-brown colour forming brittle tears known as Myrrh.

My main use for this oil is in the treatment of slow healing wounds such as ulcers. I have also found it useful for boils when blended with Lavender or Tea Tree. I have used it with some success on chapped skin brought on by weather conditions.

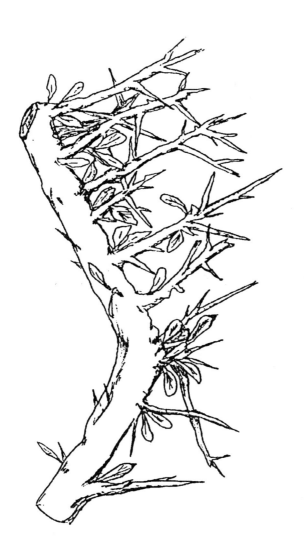

MYRRH

NEROLI

Note	Middle/Base
Botanical Name	Citrus Aurantium/Vulgaris
Family	Rutaceae
Cultivation	France, Tunisia
Part of Plant	Flowers
Extracted by	Enfleurage/ Distillation
Yield 1 Gram Oil	Equals 1000 grams base material
Constituents	**Terpenes** - Camphene, Limonene. **Nitrogen** - Indole. **Ketone** - Jasmone. **Esters** - Linalyl acetate, Methyl anthranilate, Neryl acetate. **Alcohols** - Nerol, Geraniol, Linalool, Nerolidol, Terpineol. **Acid** - Phenylacetic
Colour	Pale yellow
Aroma	Sweet, floral, but somewhat seaweed-like
Blends Well With	Most oils especially Bergamot, Lemon, Lavender, Rosemary, Sandalwood, Clary-Sage, Jasmine, Rose

| Properties | Antidepressant, Antispasmodic, Antiseptic, Aphrodisiac, Bacteriacide, Carminative, Cordial, Cytophylactic, Deodorant, Digestive, Emollient, Hypnotic, Sedative, Tonic |

MOST COMMON USES

Emotional	Anxiety, Depression, Stress, Shock, Overwork, Insomnia, Bereavement.
Skin	All skin types, especially mature, dry and sensitive
Digestive	Chronic Diarrhoea, Intestinal spasm, Flatulence
Other	Palpitations, Panic

METHODS OF USE

Bath, Massage, Inhaler, Vaporizer, Perfume

CONTRA INDICATIONS

Best avoided for younger children. Very relaxing, only use in very low dosage if a clear head is neaded.½% = 1 drop essential oil in 10ml carrier

NEROLI

Neroli is extracted from the white petals of the Bitter or Seville Orange Tree which grows up to a height of 30ft (9m). The tree originated in China but is now found throughout the Mediterranean. The best and most expensive oil comes from France, Tunisia and Sicily. It is a pale yellow liquid which darkens on exposure to light.

Neroli was first discovered in the mid 17th century and is thought to have been named after an Italian Princess , Ann Marie who lived in Neroli (near Rome); she used the oil as her favourite perfume and to scent her gloves and her bath water.

Orange flowers are worn in wedding bouquets and bridal head-dresses as a symbol of love and innocence; however this has not always been so. It is said that the perfume was once worn by prostitutes so that their customers could recognise them by their smell.

Neroli is a very useful oil, although to smell it in its pure state I think it can be off putting and strong. When blended, however, it has a most beautiful smell and is without doubt one of my own favourites.

It has many uses in Aromatherapy. I tend to use it for:- acne, anxiety, insomnia, skin care (all types), nervous tummies (especially if spasm or diarrhoea present).

Neroli is a very relaxing oil and a reputed aphrodisiac.

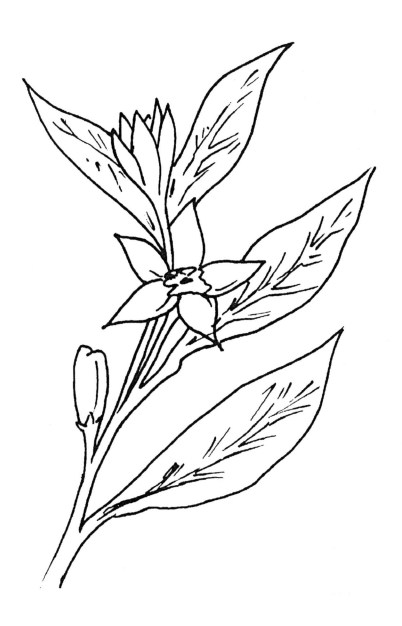

NEROLI

PATCHOULI

Note	Base
Botanical Name	Pogostemon Patchouli
Family	Labiatae
Cultivation	Malaysia, West India, Paraguay (S.E. Asia)
Part of Plant	Leaves
Extracted by	Distillation
Yield 1 Gram Oil	Equals 50 grams base material
Constituents	**Sesquiterpene** - Cadinene. **Phenol** - Eugenol. **Aldehydes** - Benzoic, Cinnamic. **Alcohol** - Patchoulol
Colour	Dark/orange brown
Aroma	Sweet/balsmic/musky
Blends Well With	Bergamot, Geranium, Lavender, Neroli, Rose, Ginger, Frankincense, Lemongrass, Sandalwood

Properties	Antidepressant, Antiphlogistic, Antiseptic, Aphrodisiac, Astringent, Cicatrisant, Cytophylactic, Deodorant, Diuretic, Febrifuge, Fungicide, Insecticide, Sedative, Tonic

MOST COMMON USES

Skin	Acne, Cracked Skins
Other	Fungal Infections, Dandruff, Obesity (induces loss of appetite), Fluid Retention

METHODS OF USE

Local, Massage, Vapouriser, Perfume

CONTRA INDICATIONS

Children
Anorexia
Prior to U.V. Sun/Sunbed

Caution   A powerful and overwhelming aroma

PATCHOULI

A native shrub of Malaysia though now cultivated in China,
India, Indonesia and the Seychelles. It grows to about 3 ft
(1 m) in height. This sturdy green, furry leaved, shrub bears
flowers that are white with the slightest hint of mauve.

The shrub is cropped about twice a year, it is another of the
soil exhausting plants so the soil needs to be well fertilised to
maintain the quality.

The Chinese, Japanese, and Malay peoples have always
respected the oil for its powers as an insect repellent. In
Victorian times leaves of the plant were placed between the
folds of cashmere shawls to protect them from moths. In India
the dried leaves or sachets were put into the beds and linen to
repel insects and bed bugs.

In view of the fact that some Patchouli is distilled under very
primitive conditions without the proper distillation receptacles
the oil may go through some changes through being exposed to
certain metals. There is no evidence to suggest that this process
has a detrimental effect on the oil's curative properties. In
order to ensure the therapeutic quality of Patchouli it should
be purchased only through a professional outlet.

I find the most use for this oil when treating the following
conditions:- abscesses, acne, cracked skin, eczema, very oily
hair, head lice, as an insect repellent in a house spray.

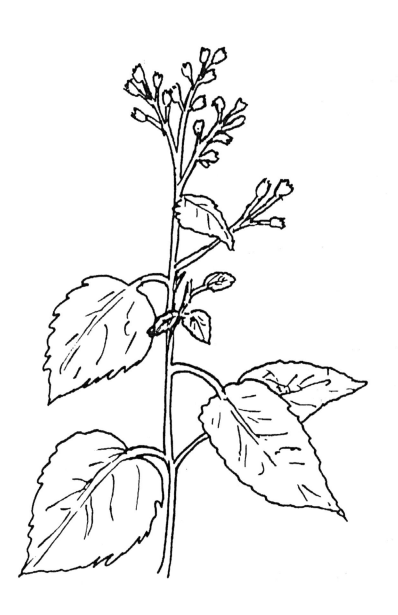

PATCHOULI .

185

PEPPERMINT

Note	Top
Botanical Name	Mentha Piperita
Family	Labiatae
Cultivation	Europe, Japan, U.S.A.
Part of Plant	Leaves/ Flowering tops
Extracted by	Distillation
Yield 1 Gram Oil	Equals 150 grams base material
Constituents	**Terpenes** - Limonene, Phellandrene. **Phenol** - Carvacrol. **Ketones** - Carvone, Jasmone, Menthone. **Ester** - Menthyl acetate. **Alcohol** - Menthol
Colour	Pale yellow, yellow, green
Aroma	Strong fresh/minty
Blends Well With	Lavender, Rosemary, Chamomile, Bergamot, Cypress, Marjoram, Mandarin

| Properties | Analgesic Antiphlogistic, Antiseptic, Antispasmodic, Astringent, Carminative, Cephalic, Cholagogue, Cordial, Decongestant, Emmenagogue, Expectorant,Febrifuge, Hepatic, Nervine,Stimulant, Stomachic, Sudorific, Vasoconstrictor |

MOST COMMON USES

Digestive	Digestive upsets, Travel sickness, Indigestion
Head	Headaches, Migraine
Other	Sinusitis, Cooling for feverish conditions

| METHODS OF USE | Compress, Local Massage, Inhalation, Vaporizer |

| CONTRA INDICATIONS | Pregnancy: - Nursing mothers, strong doses prevents sleep. Some schools of thought in the homeopathic profession believe it is best avoided when receiving their treatment as Peppermint can act as an antidote |
| | Can be irritant for Sensitive Skins |

187

PEPPERMINT

A herb that grows to about 3 ft (1 m). The leaves are serrated and hairy. Pale purple flowers appear from July to September. Various mint species hybridize naturally and peppermint is thought to be a hybrid of Mentha Aquatica (Water Mint) and Mentha Spicata (Spearmint).

A native of the Mediterranean it is also cultivated in the U.S.A. and Japan. The first recordings of peppermint cultivation in England were in 1750. Peppermint was known to the ancient Egyptians, Greeks and Romans.

The Hebrews used the oil in their perfumes which may well have been because of its reputation as an aphrodisiac.

I have found most use for the oil when dealing with digestive problems, abdominal cramps, diarrhoea and constipation.

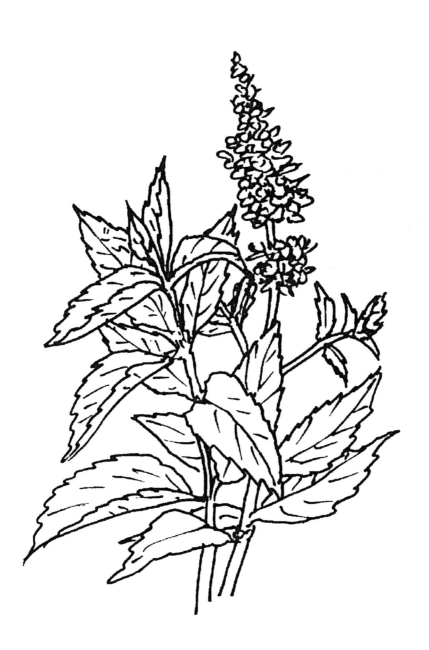

PEPPERMINT

ROSE

Note	Middle/Base
Botanical Name	France, Morocco - Rose Centifolia Bulgaria - Rosa Damascena (Otto)
Family	Rosaceae
Cultivation	Bulgaria, Morocco, France
Part of Plant	Flowers
Extracted by	Enfleurage/ Distillation
Yield 1 Gram Oil	Equals approximately 4000 grams base material
Constituents	**Terpene** - Myrcene. **Phenol** - Eugenol. **Alcohol** - Citronellol, Geraniol, Farnesol, Nerol. **Acid** - Geranic
Colour	Pale/yellow, orange/ brown, orange/green
Aroma	Rich floral
Blends Well With	Many oils especially Bergamot, Clary-Sage, Geranium, Jasmine, Patchouli, Sandalwood, Lavender, Chamomile

Properties   Antidepressant,
                              Antiphlogistic, Antiseptic,
                              Antispasmodic, Aphrodisiac,
                              Astringent, Bacteriacide,
                              Cholague, Diuretic,
                              Detoxicant, Emmenagogue,
                              Haemostatic, Hepatic,
                              Laxative, Sedative,
                              Splenetic, Stomachic,
                              Tonic, Vasoconstrictor

MOST COMMON USES   Regulating female cycle,
                              Post-natal depression,
                              Grief, Skin care (all types).
                              Rose oil is often considered
                              to be the feminine oil
                              suitable for all female
                              related problems

Under normal circumstances this oil should be used in :
                              ¼% = 1 drop - 20 ml Carrier
                              ½% = 1 drop - 10 ml Carrier
                              1% = 1 drop -   5 ml Carrier

METHODS OF USE   Bath, Compress, Massage,
                              Skin treatment products,
                              Vapouriser, Perfume

CONTRA INDICATIONS   Pregnancy

ROSE

The Rose hardly needs description. It is cultivated throughout the world (originally native to the Orient) growing on its thorny shrubs. The Damask Rose (Rosa damascena), for example, has leaves which are glossy on top and hairy underneath. It has small pink, white or red flowers arranged in coryubs (pendicles are different lengths so all flowers are the same level at the top, the outer flowers opening first).

The Rose has been prized throughout history for the colour and shape of the bloom but above all for the nature of its scent. The ancient Egyptians used roses in religious ceremonies. Roses have been found in the tombs next to the mummies.

The art of distilling Rose oil originated in Persia. The Persian warriors adorned their shields with red roses (the symbol of Persia at the time). The Romans hung roses from the ceilings during banquets and wore them to protect themselves from drunkenness (they drank Rosewater for the same purpose).

During the 17th century Bulgaria began the commercial production of Rose oil. The Bulgarians were for some considerable time the world's main producers, though Morocco and Turkey now produce vast quantities.

Rose Otto oil is the more expensive but also the more effective in therapy. The reason for the expense is twofold; firstly the low yield of essential oil from roses (100 times less than the average yield from other plants), secondly the Rose blooms for just 30 days and needs to be hand picked in the early morning during July and August. Sunshine evaporates the oil from the flower so the oil content drops. When the roses have been collected the flowers must be processed within 24 hours.

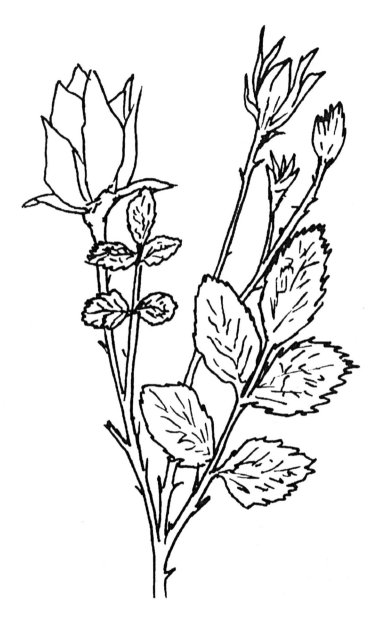

ROSE

ROSEMARY

Note	Middle
Botanical Name	Rosmarinus Officinalis
Family	Labiatae
Cultivation	France, Spain, Tunisia
Part of Plant	Flowering tops and leaves
Extracted by	Distillation
Yield 1 Gram Oil	Equals 70 grams base material
Constituents	**Terpenes** - Camphene, Pinene. **Sesquiterpene** - Caryophyllene. **Ketones** - Camphor. **Oxide** - Cineole. **Ester** - Bornyl acetate. **Aldehyde** - Cuminic. **Alcohol** - Borneol
Colour	Pale yellow
Aroma	Fresh/camphoraceous
Blends Well With	Citrus Oils, Frankincense, Lavender, Peppermint, Cedarwood, Geranium, Ginger

Properties	Analgesic, Antidepressant, Antirheumatic, Antiseptic, Antispasmodic, Astringent, Bactericide, Carminative, Cephalic, Cholagogue, Cicatrisant, Cordial, Digestive, Diuretic, Emmenagogue, Hepatic, Hypertensive, Nervine, Rubefacient, Stimulant, Sudorific, Tonic, Vulnerary

MOST COMMON USES

Digestive	Constipation, Liver/Gall bladder
Head	Poor memory Hair Loss
Muscular - Joints	Aches & pains, Arthritsis, Rhumatism
Respiratory	Asthma, Chronic Bronchitis
METHODS OF USE	Bath, Compress, Massage, Vapouriser, Inhalation (from hankie)
CONTRA INDICATIONS	Pregnancy High Blood Pressure Epilepsy

ROSEMARY

An evergreen shrub which grows to about 3 ft (1m) high, it is native to the Mediterranean region but is cultivated widely elsewhere.

The plant has a pleasant camphor-like smell and flowers from May to August. The stem is woody and branched, the leaves linear, about 1.5cm to 2.5 cm long with resolute margins (bent back at the edges). The leaf is green on top with a whitish underneath. Flower colour is a bluish-lilac.

My main use for this oil is for mental fatigue and local areas of aches and pains

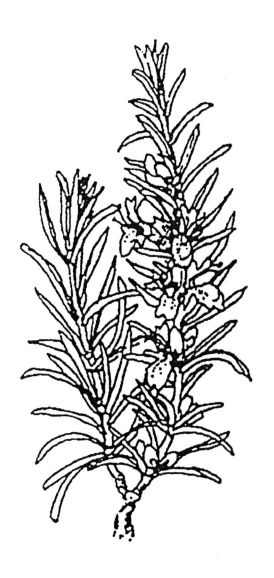

ROSEMARY

SANDALWOOOD

Note	Base
Botanical Name	Santalum Album
Family	Santalaceae
Cultivation	East India
Part of Plant	Heart Wood
Extracted by	Distillation
Yield 1 Gram Oil	Equals 25 grams base material
Constituents	**Sesquiterpene -** Santalene. **Aldehyde -** Furfural. **Alcohol -** Santalol
Colour	Pale/dark yellow
Aroma	Rich woody
Blends Well With	Black Pepper, Cypress, Neroli, Bergamot, Lemon, Frankincense, Ylang-Ylang, Lavender, and many others
Properties	Antidepressant, Antiphlogistic, Antiseptic, Antispasmodic, Aphrodisiac, Astringent, Bechic, Carminative, Diuretic, Emollient, Expectorant, Sedative, Tonic

Most Common Uses

Emotional	Nervous Tension, Depression, Insomnia
Digestive	Diarrhoea, Nausea, Colic
Skin Care	All types
Respiratory	Catarrh, Bronchitis
Other	Cystitis

Methods of Use

Bath, Compress, Massage, Vapouriser, Perfume

Contra Indications

It is an aphrodisiac so should not be used for some states of lonelines (grief) or loss of a partner

SANDALWOOD

Sandalwood is a small evergreen tree which takes approximately 50 years to reach full maturity at which point it will have reached a height of 50 ft (15m). The young grey/white trunk varies in colour as the tree matures, finally becoming yellow/orange colour. The many slender branches have oval, leathery leaves and small, pinky purple flowers.

This lovely tree starts life as a semi-parasite germinating from the black seeds of the mother tree. Roots attach themselves to nearby trees or bushes and for the next seven years the young tree depends on its host for nourishment (eventually causing it to die); at which stage the new tree can survive and grow on its own. Sandalwood must be at least 30 years of age before it can be cut down to produce oil. The oil is obtained mainly from the heart wood though some is also produced from the roots. A fully grown tree can yield up to 200 kg (400lb) of oil.

Sandalwood was used by the Egyptians both in medicine and embalming. The Indians used it for skin infections, abscesses etc. In 1868 Dr. Henderson (a Glaswegian doctor) mentioned its benefits for Blennoragia (discharge of mucus). This research was later confirmed by no less than three French doctors. During this period Sandalwood was used mainly for general urinary problems. In China it was used for stomach ache.

Although the tree has had about 4000 years of use many therapists are now concerned about the increased demand for the oil in the cosmetic and perfumery business; which in turn is causing vast areas to be robbed of trees.

Sandalwood will always be a favourite oil but my love of nature and my alarm at present day destruction limits my use of this oil to rare occasions.

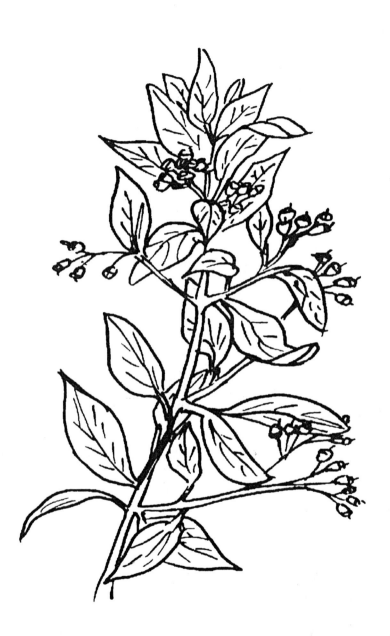

SANDALWOOD

TANGERINE

Note	Top/Middle
Botanical Name	Citrus Reticulata
Family	Rutaceae
Cultivated	China, USA, Sicily
Part of Plant	Peel
Extracted by	Expression
Yield 1 Gram Oil	Equals 150 grams of base material
Constituents	**Terpene** - Limonene. **Sesquiterpene** - Cadinene. **Aldehyde** - Citral. **Alcohols** - Citronellol, Linalool
Colour	Golden
Aroma	Tangy/ slightly sweet
Blends Well With	All oils

Properties	Antispasmodic, Cholagogue,Cytophylactic, Digestive, Sedative, Tonic
MOST COMMON USES	Depression, Convalescence, Digestion, PMT, All skin types, Children
Other	Blending- Add 1% to the floral mix makes a pleasing, less heavy, heady smell (flower oils used alone can be overpowering)
METHODS OF USE	Bath, Compress, Massage, Vapouriser
CONTRA INDICATIONS	Do not use prior to skin exposure to ultra violet (sun or sunbed)

TANGERINE

The Tangerine is very similar to the Mandarin. A native of
China, it was brought to America in the mid-19th century.

The fruit, which is smaller than an orange, is very similar to
the mandarin though more orange in colour with no pips.

I use the oil as I would Mandarin :

Children,
People convalescing,
New mothers,
All skin types,
Blending with other oils, especially the heavy florals to make
less heavy, heady oils.

Considered by some therapists to be the most suitable oil for
use in pregnancy.

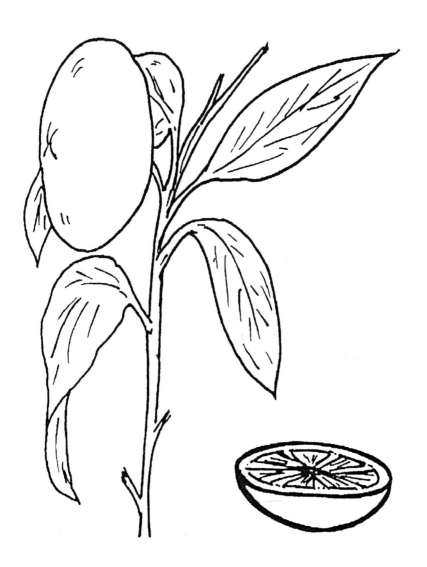

TANGERINE

205

THYME

Note	Top/Middle
Botanical Name	Thymus Vulgaris
Family	Labiatae
Cultivation	Mediterannean
Part of Plant	Flowering tops
Extracted by	Distillation
Yield 1 Gram Oil	Equals 100 grams base material
Constituents	**Terpenes** - Terpinene, Cymene. **Sesquiterpene** - Caryophyllene. **Phenols** - Thymol, Carvacrol. **Alcohols** - Borneol, Linalool
Colour	Red - First stage distillation White - Second stage distillation (Much more pure)
Aroma	Sweetish, strong herbal.
Blends Well With	Bergamot, Chamomile, Cedarwood, Juniper, Melissa, Rosemary, Tea-Tree

| Properties | Antirheumatic, Antiseptic, Antispasmodic, Aphrodisiac, Bacteriacide, Bechic, Carminative, Cicatrisant, Diuretic, Emmenagogue, Expectorant, Hypertensive, Insecticide, Stimulant, Tonic, Vermifuge |

MOST COMMON USES

Emotional	Concentration, Memory, Depression, Exhaustion,
Respiratory	Bronchitis, Tonsillitis
Circulatory	Low blood pressure
Other	Arthritic Swelling, Rheumatism, Gout

METHODS OF USE

Local Massage, Vapouriser

CONTRA INDICATIONS

Pregnancy, High blood pressure, Epilepsy, Can be a skin and mucous membrane irritant, Toxicity possible with over use

THYME

There are 3,000 species of Thyme; it is believed all or most originated from wild Thyme, a perennial evergreen shrub which grows to a height of 11" -18" (45cm). The Thyme shrub has small oval leaves, a woody root and branched upright stems. The flowers vary in colour from white or pale pink through to purple and deep red. Thyme also varies in scent from caraway or orange to mint.

Thyme has a long history; myth has it that the herb was born from the tears of Helen of Troy. Egyptians used it in the embalming process and in the days of epidemics judges carried sprigs into the courtroom to ward off infection.

Thyme is a powerful oil and should therefore be used with caution. The white oil is a purified version of the red oil. The professional therapist should use only the white oil.

My main use for this oil is in the treatment of Rheumatism and Arthritis.

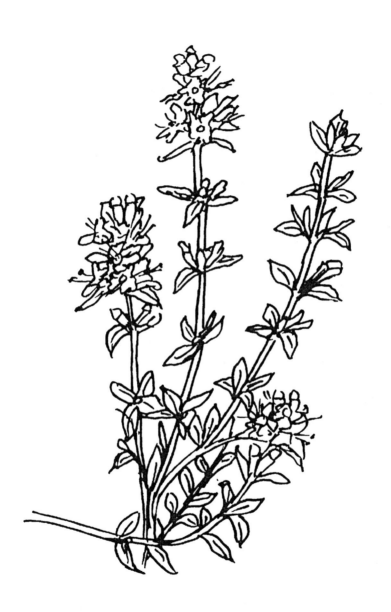

THYME

TEA-TREE

Note	Top
Botanical Name	Melaleuca Alternifolia
Family	Myrtaceae
Cultivation	Australia
Part of Plant	Leaves
Extracted by	Distillation
Yield 1 Gram Oil	Equals 90 grams base material
Constituents	**Terpenes** - Cymene, Pinene, Terpinene. **Oxide** - Cineole. **Alcohol** - Terpinenol
Colour	Yellow
Aroma	Camphor-like/balsmic
Blends Well With	Few oils. Best with Lavender, Lemon, Cypress, Rosemary, Mandarin, Chamomile
Properties	Antibiotic, Antifungal, Antiseptic, Antiviral, Bactericide, Balsamic, Cicatrisant, Cytophylactic, Expectorant, Fibrifuge, Fungicide, Insecticide, Immuno-Stimulant, Sudorific, Tonic.

MOST COMMON USES

Digestive   Gastro enteritis

Head   Mouth wash, Cold sores,
                                   Dandruff

Respiratory   Sinusitis, Bronchitis

Skin   Candida, Insect bites,
                                   Acne, Verruca, Athlets
                                   foot, Warts, Chicken Pox,
                                   Shingles, Boils, Rashes

Other   Insect repellant, Household
                                   spray when Flu is about

METHODS OF USE   Bath, Compress, Massage,
                                   Vapouriser, Alcohol Base

CONTRA INDICATIONS   Do not use this oil on very
                                   sensitive skins without first
                                   testing. Always blend
                                   before using in the bath

TEA-TREE

A small tree (Melaleuca Alternifolia) native to Australia it grows to about 20 ft (6-7m). It is similar in appearance to the Cypress with needle-like leaves and creamy-yellowish flowers. The Tea-Tree has remarkable powers of recuperation, if it is chopped down to the stump it will grow again very quickly.

The oil is obtained from the leaves and is one of the more valuable oils for treating infections and a variety of skin conditions.

The oil has a history with the aboriginal people of Australia and was one of the bush remedies used by early settlers. Tea-Tree was a remedy in the first aid kits of the Australian army and navy during the Second World War. After the war however, progression in the use of the oil slowed down and it was not until the early 70's that Tea-Tree returned to the forefront of essential oil awareness. It is now a most valued oil in Aromatherapy, though for some it may be a skin irritant.

For me Tea-Tree is a very necessary oil being anti-bacterial, anti-viral and anti-fungal. I use Tea-Tree for the following conditions: Athlete's foot, thrush (candida), warts/verrucae, herpes simplex (cold sores), shingles, chickenpox, acne, aids.

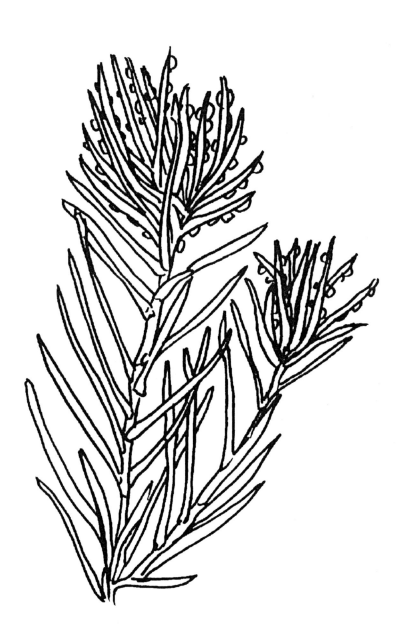

TEA-TREE

YLANG-YLANG

Note	Middle/Base
Botanical Name	Cananga Odorata
Family	Anonaceae
Cultivation	Madagascar, Java, Sumatra, Comores
Part of Plant	Flowers
Extracted by	Distillation
Yield 1 Gram Oil	Equals 100 grams base material
Constituents	**Terpene** - Pinene. **Sesquiterpene** - Cadinene. **Phenols** - Eugenol, Safrol. **Ester** - Benzyl acetate. **Alcohols** - Farnesol, Geraniol, Linalool. **Acid** - Benzoic
Colour	Pale yellow
Aroma	Spicy/floral
Blends Well With	Sandalwood, Jasmine, Bergamot, Lemon Frankincense, and many more
Properties	Antidepressant, Antiseptic, Aphrodisiac, Hypotensive, Sedative

MOST COMMON USES

Emotional

Depression, Insomnia,
Frigidity, Tension,
Anxiety, Stress

Other

Rapid heart beat, Rapid
Breathing, High blood
pressure

METHODS OF USE

Bath, Massage, Vapouriser,
Perfume

CONTRA INDICATIONS

Low blood pressure
Eczema/Dermatitis

Important Note
Do not use in high concentrations as this can cause headaches
and nausea (½% - 1% normal use) add 1 drop of Tangerine or
Mandarin to your blend to give a less heavy odour.

YLANG-YLANG

A native of the tropics, especially Indonesia, Madagascar and the Philippines, the Ylang-Ylang tree grows to 66 ft (20 m). The branches bend slightly downwards showing large sweet scented yellowish-white flowers and huge, oval shiny leaves. The wild Ylang-Ylang blossom has very little aroma.

The best quality oil comes from the Philippines but unfortunately oils from this area seem to be on the decline and an inferior quality oil from a slightly different tree which grows abundantly in Java is being sold as Ylang-Ylang, or as an alternative for Ylang-Ylang and is known only as Cananga.

Ylang-Ylang was first mentioned in the 17th century by an English botanist John Ray. It was used in a hair oil known as Macassar in Victorian times. One thing the famous hair oil did was to stain chair and sofa backs so much that washable covers, called Antimacassars, were devised for the furniture.

In the treatment of my clients I have found Ylang-Ylang most useful for the following conditions : Depression; PMS; menopausal symptoms; anxiety; shock; frigidity; anger; high blood pressure and rapid heartbeat.

Like Jasmine, Rose and Sandalwood, Ylang-Ylang is considered to be an aphrodisiac.

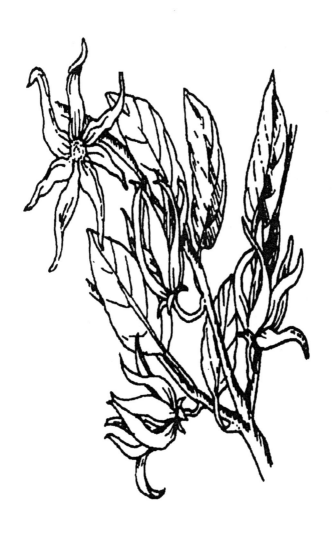

YLANG-YLANG

DIRECTORY OF DEFINITIONS AND INDEX OF PROPERTIES

A memory jogger or students

Analgesic
Reduces Pain:

Bergamot	Black Pepper
Chamomile	Cajuput
Eucalyptus	Geranium
Ginger	Lavender
Marjoram	Peppermint
Rosemary	

Antiallergenic
Reduces allergic sensitivity:

Chamomile   Melissa

Anticonvulsive
Relieves convulsions:

Chamomile	Clary Sage
Lavender	

Antidepressant
Helps lift the mood:

Bergamot	Chamomile	Grapefruit
Clary Sage	Geranium	Pettigrain
Ginger	Jasmine	Sandalwood
Lavender	Lemongrass	
Melissa	Neroli	
Patchouli	Rose	
Rosemary	Ylang Ylang	

Antiemetic
Helps to prevent vomiting:
Chamomile   Ginger

Antirheumatic
Helps relieve the symptoms of rheumatism:
Cajuput   Cypress
Eucalyptus   Jasmine
Juniper   Lavender
Lemon   Rosemary
Thyme

Anti-Inflammatory
Reduces inflammation:
Bergamot   Calendula
Chamomile   Lavender
Myrrh

Antiphlogistic
Counteracts inflammation:
Chamomile   Clary Sage
Eucalyptus   Fennel Sweet
Lavender   Patchouli
Peppermint   Rose
Sandalwood

Antipruritic
Eliminates itching:
Chamomile   Lemon

Antineuralgic
Helps relieve neuralgic symptoms:
Cajuput   Lemon

Antiscorbutic
Counteracts the effects of scurvy:
Ginger   Lemon

Antiseptic
Prevents or combats bacterial infection:
All essential oils but most effective are:

Bergamot	Eucalyptus	Ginger
Juniper	Lavender	Lemon
Rosemary	Sandalwood	Lemongrass
Tea-Tree	Black Pepper	Patchouli
Marjoram	Ylang-Ylang	

Antispasmodic
Relieves smooth-muscle spasm:

Black Pepper	Cajuput	Neroli
Clary Sage	Cypress	Rose
Eucalyptus	Fennel Sweet	Peppermint
Jasmine	Juniper	Rosemary
Lavender	Mandarin	Sandalwood
Marjoram	Melissa	Tangerine
Thyme		

Antitoxic
Counteracts poisoning:
Black Pepper

Antiviral
Inhibits growth/activity of viruses:
Eucalyptus   Lavender
Tea-Tree

Aperitif
Ginger

Aphrodisiac (Anaphrodisiac opposite of Aphrodisiac)
Increases sexual response:
Black Pepper	Ginger	Sandalwood
Jasmine	Neroli	Thyme
Patchouli	Rose	Ylang Ylang
Clary Sage		

Anaphrodisiac
Decreases sexual response:
Marjoram

Astringent
Tightens tissues:
Cedarwood	Cypress	Sandalwood
Frankincense	Geranium	Rose
Juniper	Lemon	Rosemary
Myrrh	Patchouli	Peppermint

Bactericide
Kills bacteria:
Eucalyptus	Lavender	Thyme
Lemon	Lemongrass	Tea-tree
Neroli	Rose	Bergamot
Cajuput	Juniper	Rosemary

Balsamic
Qualities of a restorative balm (Healing):
Cajuput	Clary Sage
Tea-Tree	

Bechic
Eases coughing:
Lavender	Sandalwood
Thyme	

Carminative
Prevents/relieves flatulence:

Benzoin	Black Pepper	Marjoram
Clary Sage	Ginger	Melissa
Juniper	Lavender	Neroli
Lemon	Lemongrass	

Cephalic
Clears the mind
Stimulates mental activity:

Basil	Marjoram
Rosemary	Peppermint

Cholagogue
Stimulates the flow of bile:

Lavender	Mandarin	Rosemary
Peppermint	Rose	Tangerine
Chamomile		

Citatrisant
Promotes formation of scar tissue:

Cajuput	Cypress	Patchouli
Eucalyptus	Geranium	Thyme
Juniper	Lavender	Tea-Tree
Lemon	Rosemary	

Cordial
Generally invigorating and stimulating:

Lavender	Marjoram
Melissa	Neroli
Peppermint	Rosemary
Tea-Tree	

Cytophylactic
Cell regenerator:

Geranium	Lavender	Patchouli
Mandarin	Neroli	Tea-Tree
Tangerine		

Decongestant
Relieves congestion:

Cajuput	Eucalyptus
Lavender	Peppermint

Deodorant
Reduces odour:

Benzoin	Clary Sage	Bergamot
Cypress	Eucalyptus	Petitgrain
Geranium	Lavender	Rosewood
Lemongrass	Neroli	Patchouli

Detoxicant
Helps cleanse body of impurities:

Black Pepper	Fennel Sweet
Juniper	Lavender

Digestive
Aids digestion of food:

Bergamot	Black Pepper
Clary Sage	Frankincense
Grapefruit	Mandarin
Marjoram	Melissa
Neroli	Rosemary

223

Depurative
Assists in effecting purification:
Rose

Diuretic
Increases production of urine:

Benzoin	Black Pepper	Rosemary
Chamomile	Cedarwood	Sandalwood
Cypress	Eucalyptus	Thyme
Fennel Sweet	Frankincense	Patchouli
Geranium	Juniper	Rose
Lavender	Lemon	Lemongrass

Emmenagogue
Encourages menstruation:

Basil	Clary Sage	Chamomile
Fennel Sweet	Juniper	Myrrh
Lavender	Marjoram	Peppermint
Rose	Rosemary	Thyme

Emollient
Skin or mucous membrane softener:

Chamomile	Cedarwood	Mandarin
Jasmine	Lemon	Neroli
Sandalwood		

Expectorant
Helps expulsion of phlegm:

Benzoin	Cajuput	Bergamot
Cedarwood	Eucalyptus	Peppermint
Fennel Sweet	Ginger	Sandalwood
Marjoram	Myrrh	Thyme
Tea-Tree		

Febrifuge
Reduces fever:

Bergamot	Black Pepper	Ginger
Cajuput	Chamomile	Lemon
Cypress	Eucalyptus	Melissa
Patchouli	Peppermint	Tea-Tree

Fungicide
Kills or inhibits growth of yeast, moulds, etc:

Calendula	Lavender
Lemon Grass	Myrrh
Patchouli	Tea-Tree

Haemostatic
Checks bleeding:

Cypress	Geranium
Lemon	Rose

Hepatic
Strengthens liver:

Chamomile	Cypress
Lemon	Peppermint
Rose	Rosemary

Hypertensive
Raises blood pressure:

Hyssop	Rosemary	Thyme

Hypnotic
Induces sleep:
Chamomile   Lavender
Marjoram   Neroli
Ylang Ylang   Rosewood

Hypotensive
Lowers blood pressure:
Marjoram   Ylang-Ylang   Clary Sage
Lavender   Melissa

Immuno-Stimulant
Strengthens the body's defence system to infection:
Lavender   Tea-Tree

Insecticide
Repels insects:
Cajuput   Cedarwood
Cypress   Eucalyptus
Geranium   Juniper
Lemon   Lemongrass
Patchouli   Thyme
Tea-Tree

Laxative
Promotes bowel evacuation:
Black Pepper Ginger
Lemon   Marjoram
Rose

Nervine
Strengthens the Nervous System:

Chamomile	Clary Sage	Peppermint
Juniper	Lavender	Rosemary
Marjoram	Melissa	

Parturient
Promotes and eases labour:

Clary Sage	Jasmine	Juniper

Rubefacient
Produces warmth and redness to the skin:

Black Pepper	Eucalyptus	Rosemary
Ginger	Juniper	

Sedative
Calming action on the Nervous System:

Benzoin	Chamomile	Sandalwood
Cedarwood	Clary Sage	Tangerine
Cypress	Frankincense	Ylang-Ylang
Jasmine	Mandarin	Juniper
Marjoram	Melissa	Lavender
Myrrh	Neroli	Bergamot
Patchouli	Rose	

Splenetic
Tonic for the spleen:

Chamomile	Lavender
Rose	

Stomachic
Stomach stimulant:

Black Pepper   Ginger

Stimulant
Increases activity of the body or organ:

Black Pepper	Cajuput	Geranium
Eucalyptus	Ginger	Tea-Tree
Grapefruit	Juniper	Thyme
Lemongrass	Peppermint	Rosemary

Sudorific
Promotes Sweating:

Cajuput	Chamomile	Lavender
Ginger	Juniper	Rosemary
Peppermint	Tea-Tree	

Tonic
Strengthens the body or organ:

Basil	Black Pepper	Sandalwood
Chamomile	Cedarwood	Tangerine
Clary Sage	Cypress	Thyme
Geranium	Ginger	Lavender
Grapefruit	Juniper	Frankincense
Lemon	Lemongrass	Tea-Tree
Mandarin	Marjoram	Rose
Melissa	Myrrh	Rosemary
Neroli	Patchouli	

Uterine
Tonic action on the womb:

Clary Sage	Jasmine	Rose
Melissa	Myrrh	

Vasoconstrictor
Helps small blood vessels contract:

Chamomile	Cypress	Geranium
Peppermint	Rose	

Vasodilator
Helps small blood vessels expand:
Marjoram

Vulnerary
Helps wounds to heal:

Benzoin	Chamomile	Myrrh
Eucalyptus	Geranium	Tea-Tree
Juniper	Lavender	Marjoram
Rosemary		

THE MAJOR PROPERTIES OF ESSENTIAL OILS

A MEMORY JOGGER FOR STUDENTS

Basil

Cephalic	Emmenagogue
Tonic	Sudorific

Benzoin

Diuretic	Expectorant	Carminative
Sedative	Vulnerary	Deodorant

Bergamot

Analgesic	Antidepressant	Digestive
Anti-Inflammatory	Antiseptic	Bactericide
Deodorant	Expectorant	Febrifuge
Sedative	Vulnerary	

Black Pepper

Analgesic	Antiseptic	Digestive
Antitoxic	Antispasmodic	Aphrodisiac
Carminative	Detoxicant	Febrifuge
Rubefacient	Diuretic	Laxative
Stimulant	Stomachic	Tonic

Cajuput

Bactericide	Balsamic	Analgesic
Febrifuge	Antirheumatic	Stimulant
Decongestant	Sudorific	Antineuralgic
Antispasmodic	Citatrisant	Expectorant
Insecticide		

Calendula

Anti-inflammatory	Fungicide

Chamomile

Analgesic
Diuretic
Hepatic
Nervine
Tonic
Vulnerary
Anticonvulsive
Anti-inflammatory

Antidepressant
Emmenagogue
Hypnotic
Sudorific
Vasoconstrictor
Splenic
Antiallergenic

Cholagogue
Febrifuge
Antiphlogistic
Emollient
Sedative
Antipruritic
Antiemetic

Cedarwood

Astringent
Insecticide
Tonic

Diuretic
Sedative

Emollient
Expectorant

Clary Sage

Antidepressant
Emmenagogue
Uterine
Digestive
Parturient
Tonic

Aphrodisiac
Hypotensive
Balsomic
Anticonvulsive
Antispasmodic

Deodorant
Sedative
Carminative
Nervine
Antiphlogistic

Cypress

Astringent
Hepatic
Febrifuge
Antirheumatic
Insecticide

Deodorant
Citatrisant
Haemostatic
Tonic

Diuretic
Vasoconstrictor
Sedative
Antispasmodic

Eucalyptus

Antiseptic
Deodorant
Febrifuge
Stimulant
Diuretic
Antispasmodic

Antiviral
Expectorant
Rubefacient
Vulnerary
Insecticide
Citatrisant

Bactericide
Analgesic
Antirheumatic
Decongestant
Antiphlogistic

231

Frankincense

Astringent	Diuretic	Sedative
Tonic	Digestive	

Fennel Sweet

Antophlogistic	Antispasmodic	Detoxicant
Diuretic	Emmenagogue	Expectorant

Geranium

Antidepressant	Diuretic	Astringent
Stimulant	Tonic	Vulnerary
Citatrisant	Cytophylactic	Analgesic
Deodorant	Haemostactic	Insecticide
Vasoconstrictor		

Ginger

Analgesic	Antiemetic	Antiseptic
Antiscorbutic	Aperitif	Aphrodisiac
Carminative	Expectorant	Febrifuge
Laxative	Antidepressant	Rubefacient
Stimulant	Stomachic	Sudorific
Tonic		

Grapefruit

Antidepressant	Digestive	Stimulant
Tonic		

Jasmine

Antidepressant	Emollient	Antirheumatic
Aphrodisiac	Parturient	Antispasmodic
Uterine	Sedative	

Juniper

Antiseptic	Astringent	Carminative
Bactericide	Diuretic	Citatrisant
Emmenagogue	Rubefacient	Detoxicant
Sedative	Tonic	Insecticide
Nervine	Stimulant	Antirheumatic
Antispasmodic	Parturient	Sudorific
Vulnerary		

Hyssop
Hypertensive

Lavender

Analgesic	Antidepressant	Antiviral
Anti-Inflammatory	Antiseptic	Carminative
Bactericide	Bechic	Citatrisant
Cholagogue	Cytophylactic	Cordial
Deodorant	Emmenagogue	Decongestant
Fungicide	Hypnotic	Detoxicant
Hypotensive	Immuno-Stimulant	Diuretic
Nervine	Sedative	Splenic
Tonic	Vulnerary	Antiphlogistic
Antirheumatic	Anticonvulsive	Sudorfic
Antispasmodic		

Lemon

Antiscorbutic	Antineuralgic	Antirheumatic
Antipruritic	Antiseptic	Astringent
Bactericide	Carminative	Citatrisant
Diuretic	Emollient	Febrifuge
Haemostatic	Hepatic	Insecticide
Laxative	Tonic	

Lemongrass

Antidepressant	Antiseptic	Bactericide
Carminative	Deodorant	Diuretic
Fungicide	Insecticide	Stimulant
Tonic		

Mandarin

Antispasmodic	Cholagogue	Cytophylactic
Digestive	Emollient	Sedative
Tonic		

Marjoram

Analgesic	Anaphrodisiac	Antiseptic
Antispasmodic	Carminative	Cephalic
Cordial	Digestive	Emmenagogue
Expectorant	Hypotensive	Laxative
Nervine	Sedative	Tonic
Vulnerary	Hypnotic	Vasodilator

Melissa

Antidepressant	Febrifuge	Hypotensive
Nervine	Sedative	Carminative
Cordial	Digestive	Tonic
Antiallergenic	Antispasmodic	Uterine

Myrrh

Anti-Inflammatory	Astringent	Expectorant
Emmenagogue	Fungicide	Sedative
Tonic	Vulnerary	Uterine

Neroli

Antidepressant	Aphrodisiac	Bactericide
Cytophylactic	Deodorant	Carminative
Hypnotic	Sedative	Cordial
Tonic	Antidepressant	Digestive
Emollient	Antispasmodic	

234

Patchouli

Antidepressant	Antiseptic	Aphrodisiac
Astringent	Citatrisant	Cytophylactic
Deodorant	Diuretic	Febrifuge
Fungicide	Insecticide	Sedative
Antiphlogistic	Tonic	

Peppermint

Cephalic	Cholagogue	Analagesic
Febrifuge	Hepatic	Antiphlogistic
Stimulant	Sudorific	Antispasmodic
Cordial	Astringent	Emmenagogue
Expectorant	Nervine	Vasoconstrictor
Decongestant		

Petitgrain

Antidepressant	Deodorant

Rose

Antidepressant	Aphrodisiac	Astringent
Depurative	Emmenagogue	Sedative
Tonic	Uterine	Vasoconstrictor
Bactericide	Cholagogue	Diuretic
Haemostatic	Hepatic	Antiphlogistic
Antispasmodic	Laxative	Splenic

Rosemary

Analgesic	Antiseptic	Astringent
Bactericide	Cephalic	Citatrisant
Cholagogue	Diuretic	Cordial
Emmenagogue	Hepatic	Digestive
Hypertensive	Nervine	Antidepressant
Rubefacient	Stimulant	Antirheumatic
Sudorific	Tonic	Vulnerary
Antispasmodic		

Rosewood
Deodorant   Hypnotic

Sandalwood
Antidepressant   Antiseptic   Emollient
Aphrodisiac   Astringent   Tonic
Bechic   Diuretic   Antiphlogistic
Expectorant   Sedative   Antispasmodic

Tangerine
Antispasmodic   Cholagogue   Cytophylactic
Sedative   Tonic

Tea-Tree
Antiseptic   Bactericide   Antiviral
Cytophylactic   Febrifuge   Balsomic
Fungicide   Immuno-Stimulant Citatrisant
Sudorific   Tonic   Cordial
Vulnerary   Expectorant   Insecticide
Stimulant

Thyme
Antirheumatic   Antispasmodic   Aphrodisiac
Bactericide   Bechic   Citatrisant
Diuretic   Emmenagogue   Expectorant
Hypertensive   Insecticide   Stimulant
Tonic

Ylang-Ylang
Antidepressant   Antiseptic   Aphrodisiac
Hypotensive   Sedative   Hypnotic

CLIENT CARE

The aromatherapist needs to be professional, caring, understanding and sympathetic. He/she must have the wisdom to understand when medical advice should be sought and never make claims for cures or give false hope. Neither can any guarantees be given as each blend and client is different. The professional therapist will also know that there are some oils that would never be used under any circumstances. Training will teach, all things having been considered, the most suitable oil for a particular client.

The atmosphere where the client is treated needs to be warm and relaxing with a subdued light and a subtle aroma of essential oils; the surroundings and the attitude of the therapist will have an immediate effect on the client.

When the client arrives the therapist will take his or her coat or show them where to put it. It is important for the client to be taken care of as soon as he/she arrives and that the therapist concentrates on the needs of that client. In order to do this the client has to be made to feel comfortable, be offered a seat and have the general treatment explained before the therapist starts off on a lengthy questionnaire on medical history and lifestyle. Reasons for the consultation/questionnaire should be explained to the client (e.g. a holistic approach); also the fact that blending is to suit individual needs and life-style. It should be established that there are no contra-indications (reasons why treatment cannot be performed).

The client is then asked if he/she would like to use the toilet. On returning to the treatment room the client is then asked to undress and given a bath sheet to wrap in and asked to lie face down on a couch.

Some aromatherapists ask the clients to undress completely, although naturally the client's wishes would be considered. It would not be possible to give a full body massage when the client is wearing an all in one. Personally I feel it would be easier to carry out the treatment on the back and shoulders on a female client, if she removes her bra. Where the client feels shy or embarrassed a good therapist will work by undoing the fastening and moving the straps off the shoulders. There is still a danger of either the client or the therapist getting oil on the bra (something which the therapist should explain to the client). If a pair of knickers or underpants is worn by the client they can be protected with a paper towel. Whatever the circumstance the client should always be given a modesty towel).

A Typical Consultation Card

THERAPIST'S NAME _____

Name	_____	Name of Doctor_____
Address	_____	Address_____
Telephone Number	_____	Tel Number_____
Date of Birth	_____	
Weight	_____	
Height	_____	
Occupation	_____	
Referred by	_____	
Reason for visit	_____	
Tel. No. Next of Kin	_____	
Address	_____	
Skin Type	_____	

Known Medical History

Medication _____
Previous Illnesses _____
Family Illnesses _____
Previous Operations _____
Accidents/Injuries _____
Back Problems _____
Allergies Self/Family _____
Menstrual Problems(F) _____
Marital status _____
No. of Children _____
Ages of Children _____
State of Health Gen. _____
Smoking (amount) _____
Drinking (amount) _____
Balanced Diet _____
Eating Habits _____
Regular Exercise _____
Work Routine _____
Sleep Pattern _____
Stress Prone _____
Depression Prone _____
Effects of above _____

Physical difficulties _____
Eyesight _____
Hearing _____
Posture _____

Any other condition, disorder or disease you would like to discuss_____
Are you currently receiving any other form of therapy _____
Last visit to GP_____ Reason _____
Last vistit to Hospital_____ Reason _____

CLIENT'S SIGNATURE_____ THERAPIST'S SIGNATURE_____

239

REACTIONS TO OILS

Some abnormal reactions that can occur during or
immediately after treatment
1. Nausea
2. Headaches
3. Anxiety
4. Unable to sleep
5. Itching (extreme)
6. Swelling (extreme)
7. Fainting (extreme)
Occasionally some of the above reactions may be due to the
therapist choosing the incorrect oil rather than the client's
abnormal reaction.

**Abnormal reactions can occur in anyone, especially the
following groups:**
1. Elderly
2. Children
3. Breast feeding mothers
4. Allergy sufferers
6. Asthmatics
7. Epileptics
8. Pregnancy needs special care. I personally do not use
essential oils in pregnancy. If you are considering doing so
then see a professional for advice. (Students discuss with
tutor.)

For the above, more susceptible groups : **Use oils in a more
diluted form, increasing to the desired quantity only
when convinced there is no risk.**

HINTS FOR THE THERAPIST

1. Give each client a full consultation on the first visit. Allow about half an hour for this; check medical history and life-style. On each return visit read the Record Card checking if any changes have occurred. The reason for the questionnaire should be explained, the client should be told also that the information is confidential.

2. Explain the treatment's expectations and limitations as well as what you intend to do on this visit. e.g. full body massage, treat back only, etc.

3. Ask client if he/she would like to use the toilet, show them where it is - do not create stress by sending them on a search and find mission.

4. Explain exactly which clothing needs to be removed and which can stay on. Offer to help the elderly or less able. Ask client to remove jewellery and place it in his/her bag. For security reasons the client should do this themselves.

5. Allow client to undress in privacy (if there is only one room then keep busy preparing the oils).

6. Explain to the client how you would like him/her to lie down on the couch i.e. "on the tummy, head this end." Help the client by guiding with your hand.

7. Unless weather is very warm use warm towels to cover the client.

8. Use smelling strips, blotting paper or a cotton bud to let the client smell the aroma of your mix and don't drop or drip on the clothes.

9. Make client aware that you are going to wash your hands.

10. Give the treatment. Keep to allotted time. The client may be busy; perhaps have a car in a parking bay or need to get a meal ready. He/she may like your treatments but will not return to you if you keep them over time.

11. Do not discuss politics, religion or sex. They tend to be emotive subjects. Do not gossip, ask only relevant questions in the consultation. Do not be nosey. Allow the client to sleep or talk, whichever seems best for them.

12. Remember the client is paying for your professional knowledge not to listen to your problems. Keep your own problems for your friends or go and see a professional.

13. When treatment is complete help the client off the couch, wrap in a towel and sit them on a nearby chair.

14. Go and wash your hands. On your return bring two glasses of water; one for you and one for the client. Give an explanation to the client.

15. Allow the client to dress in privacy or help if necessary. The therapist could use any free time now to complete record cards or prepare homecare preparations if required.

16. Give client a price list and any relevant publicity material.

17. Make next appointment. Try to keep to the same day and time, the client is less likely to forget. It is acceptable to remind the client to make the diary entry.

18. Throughout the treatment the client should be made to feel as though he/she is very important and special. Do not use professional jargon that the client does not understand.

19. I prefer to call people clients rather than patients. Patients conjures up pictures of illness, hospitals and doctors.

20. Always have a good knowledge of other relative therapies; otherwise you will not necessarily recognise when another therapy may be more beneficial to the client. Never contact a doctor or another therapist without client's consent.

21. Never treat beyond your skills. Never make false claims or promise cures. Be honest to yourself and others.

22. Dilution for children. Dilute ¼% - ½% to maximum of 1% depending on age. Dilute before putting into the bath. Use tea bags in the bath for babies - up to about 15 months old.

23. All oil vapours are inhaled into the lungs no matter what the method of use.

24. The professional therapist will have learned through training the oils that should not be used in Aromatherapy and the various test methods used by the industry to guarantee the quality of essential oils.

25. Membership of lead organisations is the only way for the professional therapist to be sure of any changes or additions in the uses of essential oils brought about by research and discovery.

DO'S AND DON'TS OF

AROMATHERAPY MASSAGE

THE DO'S

1   GIVE a consultation using a prepared questionnaire

2   CHECK that the chosen oils are not contra indicated to any condition/disorder on your consultation card/ questionnaire

3   CHECK your list of "Don'ts"

4   MAKE sure the room is warm

5   WASH your hands before and after treatment

6   IF playing music make sure that your client likes it and that you record the choice to avoid repetition

7   HELP client on and off the couch. If working at home a dining table with blankets on is easier to work on than the floor. The floor is easier to work on than a bed.

8.   GIVE recipient of massage a glass of water to drink when they are off the couch and dressed. The therapist should also drink a glass of water.

9. WHEN working in a clinic seeing a number of clients daily, leave the door to the treatment room open between treatments. Open the windows when the client has left.

10. WHETHER working as a professional therapist or treating the family do remember to record: the oils used, the area treated and the percentage of each oil used.

11. HOMECARE oils should have recorded on the label: Purpose of oil, Instructions for use, Date, Your own details, Telephone number, etc.

12. THE professional therapist should have a double entry of all oils supplied to clients :
        a) On the client record card
        b) A sales book for oils supplied to clients. This book should contain details of client's name, address and telephone number together with the total amount of oil blend given, base, strength and instructions for use. Cost or charge and of course the date.

13. PROFESSIONAL therapists do get client's permission if it is your intention to write to his/her GP for advice/ consent for a treatment .

14. DO use gentle strokes over varicose veins just to apply the oil to the area (not massage).

15. ASK the client to sign the questionnaire/consultation card.

THE DON'TS

1. MASSAGE infected areas

2. WHEN fever is present

3. WHEN high temperature is present

4. FOR a couple of hours after a heavy meal (especially the tummy)

5. ON an empty stomach (give a glass of fruit juice and a biscuit)

6. WHEN the recipient is under the influence of either drugs or alcohol (abuse)

7. MASSAGE OVER the area of : -
   Varicose veins (Stroke only)
   Swellings
   Inflammation
   Fractures
   Bruises
   Hernia
   Broken skin
   Recent scar tissue

8.   UNDIAGNOSED acute pain

9.   UNDIAGNOSED skin conditions

10.   IF in doubt always check with a Medical Practitioner

11.   HIGH HUMIDITY increases the permeability of the essential oil into the skin therefore the client should be advised against having an aromatherapy treatment prior to a further proposed treatment such as a turkish bath, sauna, steam bath or sunbed.

12.   MAKE sure small children do not rub their eyes whilst having an aromatherapy bath.

13.   USE skin sensitising oils on clients with allergies, Asthma, Dermatitis, Eczema, Hayfever, Skin Cancer or Melanomas.

14.   APPLY under the arms especially if any products other than washing soap is used.

15.   USE perfumed products to cleanse skin prior to aromatherapy facial.

16.   USE a strong mask on the face immediately prior to aromatherapy treatment.

Remember it is not within the skill of an Aromatherapist to make a medical diagnosis. That is the prerogative of the medically qualified or others recognised to do so.

BENEFITS OF MASSAGE

1.   Human contact
2.   Relaxes tight muscles
3.   Improves vascular and lymph flow
4.   Encourages the interchange of tissue fluid
5.   Gives a general feeling of well being
6.   Total relaxation for mind and body

In massage never use essential oils undiluted for the following reasons:

1.   No slip
2.   Highly concentrated
3.   Could overdose (due to amount that would be needed)
4.   Would cause damage (burn, rash, allergy)

SOME REASONS WHY THE CLIENT MIGHT FIND FAULT WITH A MASSAGE

Bad breath
Offensive body odour
Tobacco or stale smell on body or clothing
Being unable to see therapist's face during the treatment
Breathing into the client's face
Not showing interest in the client's problem
Nails too long scratching client
Not allowing the client to relax (talking or playing loud music)
Client may not feel therapist has taken enough care with general hygiene
Getting facial cream or oil into client's eyes
Not helping client on to and off the couch
Not explaining treatment clearly including the cost of the treatment
Taking too long with treatment
Getting products on client's clothes
Getting product on client's hair unless that is the intention

WHAT IS THE THERAPIST LOOKING FOR WHEN SHE/HE ANALYSES THE SKIN ON THE FACE/BODY?

FACE

1. Are the pores open?

2. Are there blackheads present
    chin, cheeks, nose, forehead, upper lip?

3. Are there whiteheads present
    chin, cheeks, nose, forehead, upper lip?

4. Is skin oily? Very, medium or slightly?

5. Area of oil - all over, T-zone, nose, chin, l/r cheek

6. Is the skin - thick, coarse, fine pored?

7. Is the skin dry, flaky, fine lines, areas of problems?

8. Are there broken capillaries, moles, blemishes, scars,
    pigmented areas, vitiligo?

9. What is the condition of the eyes?
    Dry, lined, dark circles, baggy underneath, crepey,
    droopy eyelids?

10.   What is the condition of the neck?
       Dry, lined, poor muscle tone, average muscle tone,
       good muscle tone (for age)?

11.   What type of oil would benefit this skin type?

12.   How many treatments?

13.   How often?

14.   What will the client expect to see as a result of the
       treatment (a. an immediate result or b. a progressive
       result)?

BODY

1.   Colour

2.   Texture

3.   Tone

4.   Blemishes

5.   Conditions

At what age do the first signs of ageing appear?
Answer - There is no age for growing old (Can become
evident at sixteen).

AROMATHERAPY AN HOLISTIC THERAPY

The word 'holistic' is taken from the Greek word 'holos' which means whole. In Aromatherpay we use it to suggest treatment that takes into account the whole person , mind, body and soul.

Plato, in his wisdom said, "The cure of the part should not be attempted without treatment of the whole".

The Greek psychologist Carl Jung wrote, "The form an illness takes can be a reflection of a mental state".

I believe that body, mind and soul are interrelated and whatever effects one will affect the whole. Therefore it is important before embarking on a treatment that we look at the life and lifestyle of our client/patient.

SOME ASPECTS OF LIVING

The professional therapist can use this guide to expand his/her own inquisitive mind in order to give maximum benefit to the client in a practical and holistic way.

1. BREATHING

Problem - Why?
Respiratory Illness
Physical damage to the Respiratory System
Common Cold
Asthma
Heart Condition

Look at the Cause
Anxiety
Emotional
Stress
Physical Conditions - Bad housing, Poor work environment,
Self employed -takes health risks, Heavy smoker

2. COMMUNICATIONS

Problem - Why?
Physical disability
Is he/she deaf?
Is he/she dumb?
Is it a difficulty to express feelings?

Look at the cause
Hereditary
Congenital
Accident
Illness i.e. malignant tumour
Surgery
Impaired mental development

Consider
Can he/she use sign language or lip read?
Can other family members use sign language or lip read?
Is there frustration?

3. EATING AND DRINKING

Problem - Why?
Mouth ulcers
Recent digestive surgery
Illness (Colitis, Crohn's disease, Ulcers, Anorexia,
Compulsive eating disorders)
Alcoholic

Look at the cause
Low income
Poor housing - shared housing, effort to get to a cooker at meal
                times
Disabled - cannot manage knobs and taps
Not educated in nutritional values
Low self esteem

Consider

Other external or internal pressures

4. CONTROLLING BODY TEMPERATURE

Problem - Why?
Elderly Person-Poor housing
> Low income
> Fear of spending money on fuel
> Risk from hypothermia

Baby-External temperature too hot or too cold

> Recognise the dangers - advise parents
> call doctor or ambulance if baby is
> showing signs for concern

5. ELIMINATION

Problem - Why?
Digestive disease or illness?
Constipation or diarrhoea induced by anxiety or stress?
Urinary disease - cystitis, incontinence (double or single)?
Is it a bed wetting child?
Is the condition caused by external or internal factors?

Considerations
Is there a medical condition?
Should the sufferer see a doctor?

6. MOVEMENT

Problem - Why?
Temporary due to joint sprain/strain or bone fracture
Is the condition psychosomatic?
Is it life threatening?
Is it degenerative?
Is it traumatic (car, bike accident) partially paralysed?

Considerations
Does he/she need referral to an Osteopath or Chiropractor?
Does he/she need hospitalisation, specialist services?

7. PERSONAL HYGIENE

Problem - Why?
Low income
Poor housing
Homeless
No bath
No hot water
Memory lapses
Mental impairment
Physical disability

8. SLEEPING

Problem -Why?
Shift work
Uncomfortable bed
Noisy neighbours
Physical pain
Pressure of work
Emotional problems

9. SEXUALITY

Problem - Why?
Infertility
Impotency
Frigidity
Illness/condition (Herpes, Thrush, AIDS)
Emotional problems
Physical problems

10. MAINTAINING A SAFE ENVIRONMENT

Problem - Why?
Low income - cannot replace damaged household equipment
Loss of smell - cannot detect smoke/fire
Physical disability - cannot mop up spillages
                    - unable to reach window catches, etc.

11. WORKING

Problem - Why?
Mentally or Physically unable
High unemployment area
Unemployment only temporary, due to accident
Suffering with depression
Housebound in wheelchair or has small children

12. DYING

Problem - Why?
Grieving for lost partner
Grieving for lost child
Grieving for lost parent
Terminally ill
Nursing a terminally ill relative, friend

The therapist will explore the possibilities as to how he/she can help in these situations :

1. By referring the client to the appropriate professional person who can deal with a particular situation.

2. By making suggestions and offering information on societies and organisations who are able to help in certain situations. e.g. housing, grants, counsellors or local organisations for the disabled.

3. The therapist should always have available an index box or book with the names and addresses of local complementary therapists and general professional organisations.

THE THERAPIST'S INDEX BOX

The therapist should always have conveniently located an index box containing useful names, addresses, telephone numbers and where applicable a named person to contact.

The list of organisations and helplines does not have to be confined strictly to conditions and complementary therapies or related fields (such as counsellers). I have found in practice it is wise to keep information on housing associations, libraries, shelters, doctors, dentists, hospitals, taxis, local police station (non-emergency numbers), RSPCA, AA, RAC, clubs for: swimming, tennis, golf, snooker, badminton, squash, fencing, bridge, ballroom dancing, bowls, cricket, gym, weight watchers, fitness centres, amateur dramatics, painting, poetry, walking, etc.

Don't forget the local mechanic and windscreen repair man, a plumber, electrician and builder. The dress hire shop and the lady who makes wedding/christening/birthday cakes.

Effort put into this when you first start your business and updated every month or so will reduce stress for both client and therapist.

Do not expect a client to remember information. Write details on a post-it sticker that has your own details stamped at the top.

WHAT IS THE HUMAN OLFACTORY SYSTEM?

The scientific name for our sense of smell is Olfaction. Smell has in the past often been considered to be the least important of the senses yet it is probably one of the oldest and may well act more directly on our subconscious than any other.

Most of the nose is concerned with processing air flow on its way to the lungs. Only a very small part of the nose and nasal cavity is taken up by the organs of smell.

The organ of smell is a little yellow patch of olfactory epithelium located in the superior aspect of each nasal cavity. Each olfactory epithelium contains about five million olfactory receptor cells surrounded by support cells. The olfactory receptor cells are bipolar neurons, each with a thin dendrite that terminates in a knob from which several cilia radiate. According to the most common hypothesis, olfactory receptor sites providing the interaction of odorants with olfactory receptors are regions of the olfactory cilia outer cell membrane formed by glycoproteins. The cilia are covered by a coat of thin mucus produced by the olfactory glands (Bowmans Glands). These secretions keep the olfactory membranes moist and serve as a solvent for the odour molecules. The mucus contains odorant binding proteins which deliver odorants to the surface of celia membranes where they bind with olfactory receptors, thus causing stimulation of olfactory neurons.

Some things you may well know about the olfactory system:

1.   In order for a substance to be smelled it must be
        volatile. In other words it must be capable of
        entering into a gaseous state. It is these gaseous
        particles that enter the nostrils.

2.   The unmyelinated axons of the olfactory receptor
        cells constitute the fibres of the 1st Cranial Nerve
        (Olfactory nerve).

3.   Our sense of smell can distinguish thousands of
        chemicals, however research suggests that we have
        only between 15 and 30 kinds of receptors. These are
        stimulated in different combinations.

4.   Pathway of Olfaction

    a. Fibres of the olfactory nerves synapse
        with mitral cells within the olfactory
        bulb.
    b. When mitral cells are activated impulses flow from
        the olfactory tract to the olfactory cortex where
        smell interpretation occurs.
    c. Olfactory tract fibres also project to the Limbic area
        of the brain where emotional aspects of the smell are
        analysed. This area is closely related to the
        hypothalmus and is also the seat of learning, memory
        and emotion.

5.   Breaths come in pairs, with the exception of twice in
        a lifetime. At birth we inhale for the first time. At
        death we exhale for the last time.

6.   We breathe about 23,000 times a day. It takes
        approximately 2 seconds to inhale and 3 seconds to
        exhale.

7.   Neurons in the nose are different to all others in the
        body in that they are replaced about every few
        months. If neurons to the brain are damaged then the
        damage is forever.

9.   Neurons in the nose are different to all others in the body in that they are replaced about every few months. If neurons to the brain are damaged then the damage is forever.

ANOSMIA

Those without sight are labelled blind, without hearing deaf. The loss of the sense of smell is known simply as anosmia. The complications and distress of such a condition are far reaching.

The loss of smell is usually the result of one or more of a number of factors. For example : Nasal cavity inflammation (caused by smoking, cold, flu), head injury, physical obstruction of the nasal cavity and olfactory mucus (e.g. polyp, genetic causes). Some brain disorders can have some effect on the sense of smell (e.g. epileptics sometimes find their sense of smell distorted).

The victim of anosmia loses not only the joy of being able to relive happy memories when receiving a luxurious rose oil massage, but the smells of danger are no longer detectable (for example the smoke filled room). The treasures and pleasures of life so many of us take for granted are denied to this almost neglected group.

OLFACTORY FATIGUE

This is in a way a form of temporary anosmia. It mostly occurs when we smell the same odour continuously over a period of time. The nose is still able to detect other odours. Sensitivity to the original smell will return if the source of the smell is removed for a little while and then returned.

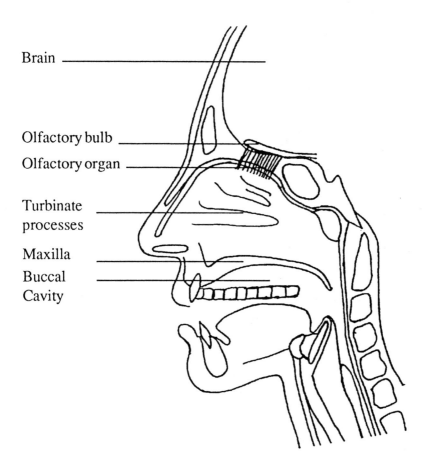

Brain

Olfactory bulb

Olfactory organ

Turbinate
processes

Maxilla

Buccal
Cavity

THE OLFACTORY SYSTEM

263

WHY IS IT ADVISABLE FOR THE CLIENT AND THERAPIST TO DRINK A GLASS OF WATER AFTER THE TREATMENT?

Aromatherapy oils are very powerful. The therapist can be subjected to many oils and over the period of a day the combination of blends can make the therapist feel heady, tired or in some cases overactive.

Drinking a glass of water after each treatment helps to prevent a build up of oils in the body and leaves the therapist feeling revived and ready for her next client.

The client should also be given a glass of water as the first step in the cleansing process from within. The water also helps to make the client feel fresh and hydrated which gives an uplifting feeling.

WINDOWS AND DOORS

CLOSING

It is advisable to close the windows and doors while giving a treatment because the room should be comfortable and warm in order for the client to relax during the treatment. If the windows and doors are left open some of the odiferous molecules from the oils will escape and therefore the impact of the oils on the Olfactory nerves in the nose of the client will be lessened.

OPENING

The windows and doors should be open between treatments in order to keep the room fresh and eliminate the build up of odours.

AREAS OF CONTRA INDICATION

PREGNANCY

When treating pregnant women I personally, do not use essential oils, except during the final stages of the pregnancy and then only in consultation with mother and midwife. My reasons for not using the oils is that I feel at present we have insufficient information from acceptable scientific research to use the oils with no element of risk; especially in the early stages of pregnancy.

In the instance of pregnancy I feel to be cautious is to be wise.

If you are considering using essential oils during **labour and delivery** please do not take a burner with you as this could be dangerous. Most hospital delivery rooms have oxygen cylinders on hand so the risk of accident is far too great. Why not use a small glass half full of water (cold is fine) into which you drop at least 4 or 5 small pieces of cotton wool, each piece having previously had 2 drops of your chosen essential oil added. As a back-up drop some oil onto a tissue and inhale when necessary; a partner can massage lower back and/or abdomen.

The following list gives a guide only and is in no way meant to be complete. If in doubt always check with a tutor or qualified therapist.

Oils considered by most therapists to be unsuitable in pregnancy are :

Basil	Cedar wood
Clary-sage	Juniper
Lavender	Marjoram
Myrrh	Hyssop
Sage	Spearmint

Oils considered unsafe to use during the first four months of pregnancy are :
  Fennel (Sweet)
  Peppermint
  Rose
  Rosemary

No oils should be used from the toxic oils list at any stage of pregnancy !

If you are not in training or a qualified therapist you should not use oils without firstly having a good knowledge of properties, uses and contra indications.

TOXIC OILS LIST

Alan Root	Elecampane	Savory
Almond (Bitter)	Fennel (Bitter)	Southernwood
Birch	Horseradish	Tansy
Bolo Leaf	Jaborandi Leaf	Terebinth
Cade	Mugwort	Thuja
Calamus	Mustard	Verbena
Camphor	Pennyroyal	Wintergreen
Cassia	Pine	Wormseed
Cinnamon Bark	Rue	Wormwood
Clove Bud	Sassafras	
Clove Leaf	Savin	
Clove Stem		
Costus		

These lists give a guide only and is not necessarily full or complete.

EPILEPSY

Do not use :
Rosemary	Fennel
Hyssop	Sage

HIGH BLOOD PRESSURE

Do not use :
Rosemary	Hyssop	Peppermint
Thyme	Sage	

Caution: When using all stimulating oils use extra caution

LOW BLOOD PRESSURE

Do not use:
Marjoram	Ylang-Ylang

THERAPEUTIC INDEX

Suitable oils and their method of use - Any one or
maximum of two oils may be used
(See Blending Guide P.65)

Abdominal Aches/Pains
Chamomile
Fennel - (Flatulence)
Peppermint
Neroli
Marjoram
Frankincense

Bath, Compress, Massage

Abrasions
Lavender
Tea-Tree
Frankincense
Neroli

Bath, Compress, Alcohol Spirit

Abcesses
Chamomile
Eucalyptus
Lavender
Lemon
Sandalwood
Tea-Tree

Compress, Bath, Alcohol spirit

Acne
Bergamot
Chamomile
Lavender
Geranium
Juniper
Melissa
Sandalwood
Tea-Tree
Thyme

Compress, Facial Steamer, Mask, Face lotion/cream

Addiction
Clary Sage
Rose
Jasmine
Neroli
Chamomile

Bath, Massage, Compress, Vapouriser

AIDS
Rose
Jasmine
Neroli
Clary Sage
Bergamot
Chamomile
Tea-Tree
Lavender

Bath, Massage, Compress, Vapouriser

Athlete's Foot
Lavender
Tea-Tree
Lemon

Bath, Compress, Cream, Alcohol

Anaemia
Chamomile
Fennel
Lemon
Petitgrain
Rosemary
Lavender

Bath, Massage, Vapouriser

Anorexia
Fennel
Bergamot
Neroli
Jasmine
Rose
Ylang-Ylang
Clary-Sage
Lavender
Chamomile

Bath, Massage, Vapouriser

Anxiety
Chamomile
Clary Sage
Frankinsense
Lavender
Rose
Geranium
Neroli
Sandalwood

Bath, Massage, Vapouriser

Arthritis
Chamomile
Juniper - If swelling is present
Ginger
Geranium
Marjoram
Rosemary
Lavender - If condition is very painful

Bath, Massage, Compress, Vapouriser

Asthma

Bergamot	Immediately prior to or directly after
Chamomile	an attack they should try one of the
Clary-Sage	following:
Cypress	Stay in moist area i.e. bathroom, or
Lavender	kitchen and add oil to water. Put the
Marjoram	drops of oil on hankie and inhale. I do
Neroli	not believe asthmatics should use
Rose	facial steamers at crucial times
Frankincense	

Bath, Compress, Vapouriser, Massage

Backache
Rosemary
Lavender
Juniper
Chamomile
Mandarin - Mix with any of the above

Bath, Massage, Compress

Bed Sores   **(Pressure sores)**
Lavender
Bergamot
Chamomile
Cypress
Geranium
Lemon

Compress, Cream

Bed wetting
Chamomile
Lavender

Bath, Massage tummy and lower back, Vapouriser

Bilious attack
Chamomile
Fennel
Ginger
Rose
Peppermint

Bath, Massage, Inhalation

273

Boils
Chamomile
Lavender
Tea-Tree

Bath, Hot compress

Bleeding
Chamomile
Cypress
Geranium
Lemon
Lavender

Compress

Blisters
Chamomile
Lavender
Lemon
Tea-Tree

Alcohol direct, Cream direct, Ice cubes

Bites
Lavender
Chamomile
Tea-Tree
Geranium
Niaouli - Neat (one drop only)

Bath, Compress, Alcohol solution, Direct application

Blood Pressure - Low (Hypotension)
Rosemary   Peppermint   - 1%
Bergamot   Black Pepper - 1%
Rose
Jasmine
Neroli
Lavender

Bath, Massage, Compress, Inhalation, Vapouriser

Blood Pressure - High (Hypertension)
Chamomile
Ylang-Ylang
Lavender
Marjoram
Rose
Neroli
Bergamot

Bath, Massage, Compress, Vapouriser

Bronchitis
Cedarwood
Cypress
Eucalyptus
Tea-Tree

Bath, Massage (chest and back), Vapouriser, Inhalation

Bruises
Lavender
Chamomile
Fennel
Geranium

Ice Compress

Burns
Lavender

Cold water then neat application. Cold compress - apply oil regularly

Bursitis
Geranium
Juniper
Rosemary
Chamomile

Bath, Compress, Massage (Rest the affected area)

Candida Albicans (Thrush)
Tea-Tree
Lavender
Myrrh
Lemongrass
Bergamot

Bath, Massage

Capillaries (broken)
Rose
Chamomile
Cypress
Calendula
Carrot

Compress, Massage (gentle), Vapouriser

Catarrh
Tea-Tree
Eucalyptus
Lemon
Lavender

Bath, Inhalation, Massage (throat, chest), Vapouriser

Cellulite
Juniper
Cypress
Lavender

Bath, Massage (strong)

Chestiness - Dry Cough
Cypress
Lavender
Eucalyptus

Massage, Vapouriser, Inhalation

Chest Cold, Infections
Tea-Tree   Ginger - For symptoms of
Eucalyptus   cold
Lavender

Bath, Massage, Inhalation

Childbirth
Jasmine

Compress, Lower back massage, Inhalation from tissue/
hankie

Chilblains
Tea-Tree   On non-infected areas
Lavender   Cypress
Chamomile   Geranium

Bath, Compress, Foot bath, Massage

Coldsore - Herpes Simplex
Tea-Tree
Lavender
Bergamot

Neat - use damp cotton wool bud to apply

Colic
Chamomile
Fennel

Bath, Abdominal massage

Colitis
Chamomile
Cypress
Geranium
Lavender
Neroli
Tea-Tree

Compress, Bath, Massage (gentle Abdominal massage)

Constipation
Peppermint
Rosemary
Juniper Berry
Fennel (sweet)
Black Pepper

Bath, Abdominal Massage (clockwise direction)

Corns
Lavender
Lemon

Local application, cover with plaster during the day

Coughing
Chamomile
Eucalyptus
Tea-Tree
Rose
Geranium
Cypress

Bath, Inhalation, Massage (chest, throat, back), Vapouriser

Cramp - leg
Geranium
Cypress
Chamomile
Rosemary

Bath, Massage, Foot bath (brisk rub)

Cramp - Abdomen
Peppermint
Geranium
Rose
Neroli
Chamomile
Bergamot

Bath, Massage, Compress

Cystitis
Bergamot
Chamomile
Eucalyptus
Juniper
Lavender
Sandalwood
Tea-Tree

Bath, Bidet, Compress, Massage (abdomen and lower back)

Dandruff
Chamomile
Clary-Sage
Cedarwood
Patchouli
Rosemary
Lavender
Tea-Tree

Lotion, Massage, Shampoo

Dental Abscess
Chamomile
Tea-Tree
Lemongrass

Massage cheek, Mouthwash with alcohol base.
Rub a piece of fresh Garlic onto the gum

Depression
Bergamot
Chamomile
Clary-Sage
Jasmine
Neroli
Rose
Sandalwood
Ylang-Ylang

Bath, Massage, Vapouriser

Dermatitis
Bergamot
Chamomile
Cedarwood
Geranium
Juniper berry
Lavender
Rosemary
Rose
Peppermint
Sandalwood

Bath, Massage, Compress

Diarrhoea
Chamomile
Cypress
Ginger
Lavender
Neroli
Peppermint
Sandalwood
Tea-Tree

Compress, Gentle Massage (abdomen) - (reduce food intake
and drink lots of water - seven pints a day)

281

Diabetes
Eucalyptus
Geranium
Juniper
Bergamot
Black Pepper
Rose
Neroli

I do not recommend
Sweet Almond as a carrier

Bath, Massage, Vapourisation

Digestive Problems
Chamomile
Fennel (sweet)
Ginger
Lemongrass

Bath, Massage, Compress, Vapourisation

Diverticulitis
Bergomot
Chamomile
Eucalyptus
Marjoram
Peppermint
Tea-Tree

Bath, Massage, Compress

Energy Depletion
Rose
Rosemary
Bergamot
Geranium

Bath, Massage, Vapourisation

Earache
Chamomile
Lavender
Tea-Tree

Blend all three oils together and massage around outside of the ear

Eczema
All oils used for dermatitis - See 'Dermatitis' (page 281)

Epilepsy
Chamomile
Cypress
Lavender
Tangerine

Bath, Vapouriser

Exhaustion
Clary-Sage
Mandarin
Lavender
Bergamot

Bath, Massage, Vapouriser, Inhale from hankie

Fainting
Peppermint
Rosemary
Neroli
Lavender

Compress, Vapouriser - Inhalation from hankie or direct from the bottle

Flatulence
Fennel
Ginger
Petitgrain
Mandarin

Bath, Compress, Massage

Fever
Peppermint
Lavender

Bath, Compress, Inhalation

Fleas
Lavender
Tea-Tree
Eucalyptus

Bath, Local direct application

Frigidity
Clary-Sage
Rose
Jasmine
Ylang-Ylang
Sandalwood

Bath, Massage, Vapouriser

Fibrositis
Chamomile
Cypress
Lavender
Juniper
Rosemary

Bath, Compress (alternate hot/cold), Massage, Vapouriser

Gallbladder - Stimulant
Lemon
Rosemary
Chamomile
Peppermint
Lavender

Bath, Compress, Massage, Vapouriser

Gout
Chamomile
Lavender
Cypress
Juniper
Ginger

Foot bath, Compress

Hangover
Rose
Rosemary
Juniper

Bath, Head and abdominal massage, Vapouriser, Inhalation
from tissue/hankie

Hayfever
Juniper

Vapouriser, Inhalation from tissue/hankie

Headaches
Chamomile
Lavender - Tension
Peppermint
Rosewood
Juniper - Allergy
Rose   - Allergy

Bath, Compress, Vapouriser, Massage

Herpes Zoster

Chamomile
Eucalyptus
Geranium
Lavender
Tea-Tree

Bath, Compress, Vapouriser

Hoarseness
Sandalwood
Lavender
Eucalyptus

Massage, Vapouriser, Inhalation from tissue/hankie

Hot Flushes
Rose
Chamomile
Geranium

Bath, Massage, Vapouriser, Inhalation from tissue/hankie

Hypertension - See High Blood Pressure

Hypotension - See Low Blood Pressure

Indigestion
Peppermint
Chamomile

Bath, Compress, Inhalation from tissue/hankie, Abdominal massage (clockwise)

Impotence
Clary-Sage
Jasmine
Peppermint
Sandalwood
Rose

Bath, Massage, Vapouriser

Insomnia
Chamomile
Lavender
Marjoram
Mandarin
Ylang-Ylang

Bath, Massage, Vapouriser

Kidney Problems
Bergamot   Cedarwood
Fennel   Frankincense
Geranium   Juniper
Sandalwood

Bath, Compress, Massage

Lice
Eucalyptus
Geranium
Lavender
Tea Tree

Head massage/shampoo, Hair spray

Ligaments - Painful
Lemongrass
Rosemary
Lavender

Bath, Local massage, Compress

Liver
Rosemary
Chamomile
Peppermint
Juniper
Lemon

Bath, Hot/Cold Compress

Lymphatic System
Grapefruit
Geranium
Fennel
Juniper
Rosemary

Bath, Massage. DO NOT give lymphatic drainage massage to patients suffering with Cancer or Aids or any serious condition of the auto immune system.

Menopause
Chamomile
Geranium
Rose
Jasmine
Lavender
Ylang-Ylang
Neroli
Bergamot
Sandalwood

Bath, Massage, Compress, Vapouriser

Memory
Basil
Rosemary
Peppermint

Bath, Massage, Inhalation

Metabolism - Sluggish
Lavender
Lemon
Peppermint
Rosemary
Juniper

Bath, Massage, Vapouriser

Migraine
Chamomile
Cypress
Fennel
Lavender
Lemon
Marjoram
Peppermint

Bath, Compress, Self massage around temples (very light)

Mosquitoes
Lavender   Lavender - Apply directly
Eucalyptus   onto bites
Lemongrass

Bath, Spray body (in either vinegar or alcohol base)

Muscle Aches
Chamomile
Lavender
Rosemary
Marjoram
Juniper

Bath, Massage, Compress

Multiple Sclerosis (M.S.)
Bergamot
Chamomile
Juniper
Peppermint
Rosemary

Bath, Massage, Compress, Vapouriser

Myalgi-Encephalomyelitis (M.E.)
Chamomile
Geranium
Grapefruit
Lavender
Neroli
Rose
Sandalwood
Tea-Tree

Bath, Compress, Inhalation, Vapouriser

Nausea
Peppermint   - Travel sickness
Spearmint   - Travel sickness
Rosewood
Chamomile
Neroli
Lavender   - with migraine

Bath, Abdominal massage, Inhalation, Vapouriser

Neuralgia
Peppermint
Chamomile
Lavender

Compress, Gentle Massage, Vapouriser

Nettle Rash
Chamomile
Lavender

Cold Compress, Cool Bath

Nappy Rash
Lavender
Chamomile
Wheatgerm

Bath, Cream (see "Recipe" section page 324)

Obesity

Fennel   Female - Rose, Geranium
Grapefruit   Male - Jasmine, Sandalwood
Orange
Bergamot

Bath, Massage, Diffuser, Inhalation from tissue or hankie

Palpitations

Chamomile
Lavender
Neroli
Clary-Sage
Ylang-Ylang
Rose

Bath, Massage, Vapouriser

Perspiration

Cypress
Geranium
Rose

Bath, Foot bath, Massage, Alcohol-based spray

Premenstrual Syndrome
Bergamot
Chamomile
Clary-Sage
Fennel
Geranium
Lavender
Marjoram
Neroli
Rose
Ylang-Ylang

Bath, Massage, Compress, Vapouriser, Inhalation

Periods - Heavy
Cypress
Rose
Geranium

Periods - Painful
Chamomile
Marjoram
Lavender

CHECK with your GP and
then with a professional
therapist

Periods - Scanty, Late
Clary-Sage
Fennel
Rose (Regulator)
Juniper
Rosemary

DO NOT use essential oils
if there is a chance you
might be pregnant

Baths, Compress, Massage abdomen and lower back

Psoriasis
Bergamot
Chamomile
Eucalyptus
Frankincense
Juniper
Lavender
Rose
Sandalwood

Bath, Local Compress, Vapouriser

Respiratory Weakness
Cypress
Eucalyptus
Lavender
Peppermint
Tea-Tree
Rosemary

Bath, Massage, Compress, Inhalation, Vapouriser

Rheumatism
Bergamot
Chamomile
Juniper
Lavender
Marjoram
Neroli
Rosemary

Bath, Compress, Massage

Rubella
Bergamot
Chamomile
Cypress
Eucalyptus
Lavender
Sandalwood
Tea-Tree

Bath, Compress, Vapouriser

Sinusitus
Cypress
Eucalyptus
Lavender
Tea-Trea

Inhalation, Vapouriser, Facial Massage

Sprain (Joint)
Chamomile
Eucalyptus
Lavender

Compress (fold)

Strain (muscle)
Bergamot
Chamomile
Clary-Sage
Geranium
Neroli
Rose
Sandalwood

Bath, Massage, Vapouriser, Inhalation

Tension
Bergamot
Chamomile
Clary-Sage
Jasmine
Juniper
Lavender
Marjoram
Neroli
Rose

Bath, Massage, Vapouriser, Inhalation

Tonsillitis
Geranium
Chamomile
Lavender
Tea Tree

Bath, Vapouriser, Inhalation

Toothache
Chamomile
Niaouli
Tea Tree
Lavender

Massage cheek, Mouthwash solution in alcohol base

Urinary Infections
Bergamot
Cedarwood
Eucalyptus
Niaouli
Tea-Tree
Sandalwood

Bath, Bidet, Compress, Massage, Vapouriser

Varicose Veins - Legs
Cypress
Lemon
Geranium

Bath, Massage (very gentle stroking)

Varicose Veins - Haemorrhoids
Cypress
Chamomile
Geranium

Bath, Bidet, Lotion/Cream

Viral Conditions
Eucalyptus
Lemon
Tea-Tree
Melissa

Vapouriser, Local application, Inhalation

Water Retention
Cypress
Fennel
Juniper
Geranium
Grapefruit

Bath, Massage, Compress

Wounds (Infected)
Lavender
Frankincense
Tea-Tree

Compress - wash/soak, Direct application

RECIPES

MASSAGE OILS FOR SPECIFIC CONDITIONS
BLENDED IN 25 ML CARRIER

Anxiety/Depression

4 drops Clary-Sage
2 drops Patchouli
4 drops Ylang-Ylang

Apathy/Anxiety

4 drops Grapefruit
4 drops Lavender
4 drops Rosemary
            or
4 drops Neroli
4 drops Lavender
2 drops Lemon

Extreme Nervousness

2 drops Clary-Sage
2 drops Jasmine
4 drops Bergamot

Irritability

4 drops Petitgrain
2 drops Sandalwood
4 drops Chamomile

Nervous Tension/Hysteria

4 drops Neroli
4 drops Chamomile
4 drops Sandalwood

Spasticity

Local Massage of area

6 drops Ginger
6 drops Lavender
      or
6 drops Cypress
6 drops Chamomile
      or
6 drops Rosemary
4 drops Sandalwood
2 drops Chamomile

Relaxing Oils

4 drops Geranium
8 drops Chamomile
or
4 drops Rose
2 drops Tangerine
or
8 drops Lavender
4 drops Chamomile
or
8 drops Marjoram
4 drops Chamomile

Stimulating Oils

8 drops Rosemary
4 drops Bergamot
or
6 drops Peppermint
4 drops Lavender
or
8 drops Rosemary
4 drops Lemon

BATH OILS

NOTE:-BLEND BATH OIL IN VODKA, CREAM OR CARRIER OIL PRIOR TO PUTTING INTO BATH. I USUALLY BLEND BATH OILS 3 DROPS ESSENTIAL OIL TO 5ML OF CARRIER (APPROX 1 TEASPOON)

Aphrodisiac Bath

2 drops Sandalwood
1 drop Ylang-Ylang
        or
1 drop Sandalwood
1 drop Neroli

Wake-Me-Up Bath   am or pm

2 drops Rosemary
1 drop Geranium
        or
1 drops Peppermint
1 drop Rosemary
1 drop Geranium

Fluid Retention/Cellulite

1 drop Geranium
1 drop Juniper
1 drop Sweet Fennel

or
1 drops Juniper
1 drop Sweet Fennel
1 drop Cypress

Insomniac Bath

1 drop Clary-Sage
2 drops Chamomile

Total Indulgence Bath

2 drops Rose
1 drop Mandarin
      or
1 drop Jasmine
2 drops Mandarin
      or
2 drops Neroli
1 drop Geranium

TIPS FOR AN AROMATIC BATH OR SHOWER

Prepare your bath in the normal way. Do not have the water too hot as it is not good for your skin. Pour your prepared essential oil mixture into the water and swish it gently around. Now get into the bath and soak. Try twenty minutes of sheer self-spoiling luxury. Fifteen minutes will also do you the world of good.

NOTE
A maximum of 3 drops of essential oil to any bath or shower, irrelevant of the amount of base or carrier used.

You will need:
A glass or plastic measure available from a chemist shop
A carrier oil or emulsifier
Your essential oil

To dilute or emulsify your essential oil you can use one of the following base/carriers:

Oil - 5 ml for oily skin / 15 ml for dry or mature skin.

Honey - 15 ml for all skin types; as honey is very balancing and nourishing for the skin

Whipped Cream - 15 ml for all skin types

Vinegar - 5 ml for dry or mature skin 10 ml for oily, blemished skin

Vodka - 5 ml for dry or mature skin. 10 ml for oily, blemished skin

Liquid Soap - 15 ml for bath, 20 ml for shower

Brandy may be substituted for the Vodka but be warned - it does have an alcoholic smell.

Shower

Get into the shower and allow water to run over the body in the normal way for about one minute. Don't have the water too hot. Turn off the shower and apply the prepared liquid soap all over the body; then shower again.

PRODUCT RECIPES

GENERAL BASE CREAM/OINTMENT

You will need:

50 ml	Grapeseed
50 ml	Wheatgerm or suitable alternative oil
25 grams	Yellow Beeswax
125 drops	of essential oil

A large saucepan
A tall pyrex or metal jug
A spatula or long handled spoon
Some small pots/jars

If you would like a softer cream make the following blend :

70 ml	Grapeseed
55 ml	Wheatgerm
25 grams	Yellow Beeswax
25 grams	Vaseline - or instead of Vaseline use 10 ml Rose Water and 15 ml Glycerine
175 ml	Add to this mixture 175 drops of oil

Note - Vaseline offers a protective external fil.

HOW TO PREPARE YOUR MIX

Prepare a large saucepan of water and place on a stove. Into this you stand a tall jug-type pyrex or stainless steel container.

1. Add the wax to the jug
2. When wax has melted reduce the heat under the saucepan

3. Add all other ingredients, apart from the essential oil

4. Leave saucepan on the stove and stir the mix together. Do not allow the mix to boil

5. Turn off the stove and carefully remove the jug from the water

6. Wait for the mix to begin to cool and set

This shows around the edge of the pot first - as soon as setting begins pour your essential oil drops into the mix and stir all the ingredients together.

Note - if wax is grated it will melt faster.

Pour the contents of the jug into individual pots and stand these pots in a tray of cold water so they are submerged to between one third and half their height.   Alternatively surround the pots with ice.   This action speeds up the cooling process.

Seal the pots, wipe dry and label.

This cream should last for about a year especially if a clean cotton wool bud is used each time some of it is removed.

Note:
Use for localised conditions only. eg. sprains/strains, Athletes Foot, boils, frozen shoulder, acne spots on the back etc. In our ointment mix we have 175 ml of ointment and 175 drops of essential oils = 5% Essential oil blend.

SKIN CARE GUIDE

Suitable Oils for Home Preparation

Dry Skin

Rose
Chamomile
Sandalwood
Neroli
Frankincense

Oily Skin

Rose
Rosemary
Lavender
Grapefruit
Geranium

Mature Skin

Rose
Neroli
Frankincense
Sandalwood
Ylang-Ylang

Acne

Rosemary
Juniper
Lavender
Tea-Tree
Geranium

Sensitive Skins
Use no more than 1 drop to 10ml

Rose
Chamomile
Lavender

Patch test if worried

CLEANSING CREAM

You will need:
60 ml Almond oil
60 ml Rosewater
15 grams Beeswax
10 drops essential oil
A large saucepan
A tall pyrex or metal jug
A spatula or long handled spoon
A rotary whisk or fork
Some small pots/jars

Method of preparation:
Prepare a large saucepan of water into which you stand a tall
jug-type pyrex or stainless steel container.
Place the wax and oil into the jug and wait for the wax to melt
(grated wax will melt quicker).
Turn off the source of heat. Remove the jug carefully from
the saucepan.
Slowly add the Rosewater while using a rotary whisk or a
fork. Continue to add slowly and whisk until all the water has
been absorbed (do not overbeat).
Add the essential oil to the mix and stir all the ingredients
together; the handle of a long spoon can be used if a clinic
spatula is not available.
Empty the mix into small individual pots and stand them on a
tray surrounded by ice. If no ice is available then put cold
water in the standing dish/tray. When cool, seal, wipe dry and
label clearly.
Now place the pots in a cold place; they should keep for about
six to eight weeks.

SKIN TONIC

What you will need:
200 ml Bottle

80 ml	Orange flower water or Rosewater
80 ml	Filtered fresh water/tap water
10 ml	Alcohol (Vodka)
16 Drops	Essential oil

For a very oily skin use 20 ml vodka / 70 ml water.

Method of Preparation:
Blend oil into vodka
Pour into 200 ml bottle
Add floral water
Add filtered water
Label bottle
Turn bottle up and down about 10 times. Shake gently each time before use.

NOTE

Prior to an aromatherapy massage the face should be cleansed of all creams, masks, etc. . The use of a toner just before a massage should help to ensure this and avoid cross sensitization.

SKIN MOISTURISER / CREAM

What you will need :

60 ml	Almond oil
7 grams	Beeswax
15 ml	Distilled water
2 ml	Vitamin E oil
8 Drops	Essential oil

A large saucepan
A tall pyrex or metal jug
A spatula or long handled spoon
A rotary whisk or fork
Some small pots/jars

Method of preparation is exactly the same as for the cleansing cream.

NOTE
If skin is very dry or mature the moisturiser can be altered in one of two ways:

1. Instead of 60 ml Almond oil use 30 ml of Almond oil and 30 ml of Avocardo plus 1ml of Evening Primrose oil (to be added with the Vitamin E oil).

2. Use 60 ml of Jojoba oil instead of Almond or Avocado plus 1ml of Evening Primrose oil.

Either of these alternative mixtures are suitable as night creams or neck creams.

FACIAL MASK
Use Clay; it is best for cleansing (use 2 days prior to essential oil massage)

What you will need:
A small bowl or cup,
A wooden spatula or orange stick
Mask ingredients
3 Teaspoons powdered clay e.g. Fullers Earth
About 1 tablespoon of water
Essential oil
(For very greasy/oily skins use Witch Hazel instead of water)

Method of preparation:
Add 3 teaspoons of powder clay to bowl
Add water
Mix to a paste consistency
Add 1 drop of essential oil to ½ teaspoon (2½ ml) of Witch Hazel
Mix all ingredients again

If your mask is very runny then just add a little extra powder to form a paste again.

How to apply:
Apply mask to the neck and face (like painting). Avoid nostrils, lips, eyes and soft skin underneath the eye. Use a damp 1 inch (2 cm) paint brush/mask brush, this is best for the smooth application of mask. Remove the mask after five minutes for dry, mature and sensitive skins. 10 minutes for normal skins and 15 minutes for oily, acne skins. Damp facial sponges are best for mask removal. If not available then use clean face flannels.

After removal of mask :
Tone skin using damp cotton wool pads.
Moisturize skin using fingers.
If skin feels greasy blot with tissue to remove excess;
do not rub.

The professional aromatherapist may use a cream/biological
mask prior to a facial massage. Honey or Azuline is suitable
for almost any skin types. A very oily skin skin may need a
strawberry or cucumber mask.

NOTE

Prior to an aromatherapy massage the face should be cleansed
of all creams, masks, etc. . The use of a toner just before a
massage should help to ensure this and avoid cross
sensitization.

SKIN MAINTENANCE

Daily (x2 for All skin types)

| Cleanse | Tone | Moisturise | | |

Weekly (x1 for Normal, Dry, Mature)

| Cleanse | Tone | Mask | Tone | Moisturise |

Weekly (x2 for Very Oily)

| Cleanse | Tone | Mask | Tone | Moisturise |

FACIAL COMPRESS

Compresses are similar to steaming but have two advantages:
1. Control on a specific area to be treated
2. Oils used in this way are believed to be absorbed more quickly and the skin feels softer afterwards

Requirements :
2 pint bowl
4 face flannels
1 pint hot water
Essential oil

Add 2 drops of essential oil to the water
swish around
Place flannels in water, then wring out excess water
Put on the face for a few minutes
When cool repeat the process for about five times

The professional therapist with the necessary qualifications could use an Infra Red Lamp at a distance of 24 inches from the face to keep the compress warm (protecting the eyes)

Kitchen foil could be used as an alternative to Infra Red to help retain the heat

FACIAL STEAMING

The professional therapist would always establish that the client being treated does not suffer with claustraphobia. The professional will also cover the eyes with cotton wool and can regulate the distance from and volume of steam reaching the skin.

For these reasons I am more in favour of professional treatments. Home equipment usually requires that the whole face be subjected to steam and therefore areas of broken capillaries might be over stimulated. It is also not possible to protect the eyes with cotton wool and lean forward at the same time. For home use the user may like to try protecting his/her eyes by wearing swimming goggles and areas of sensitive skin/broken capillaries with a good barrier-type cream.

Benefits of steaming:
Adds moisture
Aids penetration
Cleanses the pores
Enables skins such as acne types to be treated without the possible irritation from touching with cotton buds or spatulas

Add 2 drops of oil blended in 5 ml of Vodka to the water

Allow the skin to cool prior to application of essential oil massage

Can be used prior to a mask to soften the skin
AFTERSHAVE

What you will need:
200 ml   Bottle
150 ml   Orangeflower water
 15 ml   Vodka
 10 drops of essential oil

Most suitable oils are Sandalwood, Bergamot or Cypress

Method of preparation is as for Skin Tonic

How to apply:
Splash on face and neck

Benefits:
Soothing, tightens the pores and helps prevent skin pimples, etc.

MOUTH WASH

What you will need:
250 ml Bottle (plastic for the bathroom)
250 ml Vodka
  20 Drops of Thyme
  10 Drops of Tea-Tree
  10 Drops of Fennel
  20 Drops of Peppermint

How to prepare your mix:
Add Vodka to the empty bottle
Add essential oil

How to apply:
Add 15 ml (approx. 3 teaspoons) of your mixture to half a
tumbler of water
Use as normal mouthwash
Remember to shake bottle before each use

SHAMPOO

Purchase a natural shampoo such as Chamomile. To each 100 ml add 10 drops of essential oil. Use the shampoo in the normal way. A total of two oils is recommended with the maximum being three.

Hair care index guide:

Dry Hair	**Oily Hair**	**Dandruff**
Sandalwood	Rosemary	Rosemary
Geranium	Juniper	Tea-Tree
Rose	Bergamot	Eucalyptus
Ylang-Ylang	Clary-Sage	Lavender
	Lemon (if blond)	

HEAD LICE SHAMPOO

Purchase a natural shampoo such as Chamomile. To each 100 ml add 20 drops of essential oil. Use the shampoo in the normal way. A total of two oils is recommended with the maximum being three

The oils to use :

Eucalyptus
Geranium
Lavender
Tea-Tree

Wash twice daily for one week and then twice per week for two weeks

HAND AND NAIL CARE

What you will need for basic preparation:

50 ml   Bottle
25 ml   Avocado oil
25 ml   Grapeseed

Cracked Brittle Nails
add
20 Drops   Lemon

Bitten Nails and Skin
add
10 Drops   Lavender
 5 Drops   Lemon
 5 Drops   Chamomile

Nail Fungus
20 ml   Vodka
12 Drops   Tea-Tree
 2 Drops   Lavender
Apply three times each day

Dry Hands

Use basic preparation as for Nails but use Essential Oil of:

5 Drops   Geranium
5 Drops   Chamomile
2 Drops   Rose
or instead of Rose use :
5 Drops   Frankincense

ATHLETE'S FOOT RECIPE

What you will need:
20 ml Pot bland cream

add
10 Drops Tea Tree
10 Drops Lemon

Massage into feet twice a day

or
20 ml Vodka

add
10 Drops Lavender
10 Drops Tea Tree

Massage into feet twice a day until condition improves

VERRUCA

What you will need :
20 ml Vodka

add
6 Drops Lemon
6 Drops Tea-Tree
2 Drops Lavender

Apply directly onto Verruca in the morning and cover with a plaster. Remove plaster at night and re-apply mixture. Leave uncovered overnight

NAPPY RASH

FIRST AID

Prepare a general base cream or ointment as described on page 307 or 312

To 40 ml of the base cream/ointment add :

  5 ml of Wheatgerm oil
20 Drops of essential oil = 12 of Lavender, 8 of Chamomile
  5 Drops of either Jojoba or Avocado

If you do not have the facilities to follow the recipe on page 307 or 312 then purchase a bland cream from the chemist and add the suggested oils.

REGULAR - NAPPY CHANGE CREAM

Prepare the base cream/ointment as previously described only this time increase the base quantity to 100 ml. The other quantities and ingredients should remain the same as for the 'First Aid' cream

ROOM SPRAY / AIR FRESHENER

What you will need:
100 ml plastic bottle with spray top
20 ml Vodka
80 ml Water
20 Drops Essential oil

How to prepare your mix:
Add Vodka to the empty bottle
Add 20 drops essential oil
Add the water
Put the cap onto the bottle and shake vigorously

Most suitable oils to use depends on the reason for use but you can use a mixture. I often rinse out the dregs from the bottom of the oil bottles for this purpose

To create a clean, fresh smell use Lemon or Cypress.
For floral smells use Ylang-Ylang, Sandalwood or Geranium

Why not experiment?

KEEP AT BAY

Lavender	Moths, Mosquitoes, Fleas, Flies
Lemongrass	Ticks
Peppermint	Ants

Method of use:
Spray area of habitat. Hang some ribbons soaked in essential oil from the curtain rail. Put soaked cotton wool pads in the area. For infested animals rub effected area or put a drop on the collar

USEFUL TERMS

1. **Carcinogenic**
   An agent capable of inducing cancer.

2. **Irritation Cutaneous**
   The result when a substance reacts with the skin (can be localised) depending on where substance is applied or it can be generalised, causing swelling and pain.

3. **Idiosyncratic Sensitisation**
   An abnormal reaction to a normally harmless substance. In other words it is an individual reaction rather than perhaps one of the less common reactions such as allergy to metal.

4. **Mucous Membrane**
   Composed of cells that secrete a protective mucus fluid. The name mucous membrane is given to the linings of : the Alimentary Tract, Genito-urinary Tract and Respiratory Tract.

5. **Photosensitisation or Phototoxicity**
   Reactions of skin that is exposed to ultra violet light after the application of essential oil.

6. **Sensitisation**
   Simply means allergic reaction. An intense form of irritation involving the immune system. Even small amounts of the offending agent can cause severe reactions.

7. **Acute**
Short and severe, not long drawn out or ongoing.

8. **Chronic**
Lasting, ongoing.

9. **Infusion**
A herbal preparation made by pouring boiling water on the fresh or dried herb (as for teas).

10. **Decoction**
A herbal preparation made by boiling the plant material for 10-20 minutes, starting with cold water.

11. **Maceration**
A herbal preparation made by steeping the plant material at room temperature for hours or days. The liquid may be water, alcohol, wine or oil (see below).

12. **Herbal Oil**
An oil prepared by steeping the plant material in a bland oil.

13. **Tincture**
A clear liquid prepared by macerating the plant material in alcohol, pressing and finally filtering.

14. **Essence**
A substance which naturally occurs within a plant.

15. **Essential Oil**
The result of the extraction of the essence from the plant by means of distillation.

16. **Osmosis**
Tendency of solvent to diffuse through porous partition into more concentrated solution.

17. **Gas Liquid Chromatography (GLC) Analysis**
A piece of equipment used in the laboratory to separate the vapour of a volitile mixture into its individual components. The results of the GLC are printed out by an instrument onto a sheet of paper as a series of peaks, each peak corresponding to one of the constituents of the product being analysed. For accuracy the results of the GLC analysis must be interpreted by an expert in the field.

18. **Mass Spectrometer**
An instrument coupled to the GLC which breaks up into fragments the molecules of the individual constituents of the products from which the analyst can then identify a constituent.

19. **I.R. Spectrophotometer**
An infra red instrument which gives a graph reflection of the composition of the material being tested. Each essential oil has its own characteristic print. Like human fingerprints each essential oil print is individualistic, being different from those of all other essential oils.

QUICK REFERENCE

Compress

Can be used in almost any area as it is easy to mould the material to the contours of the body including the face (small guest towels, face towels or two face flannels can be used). Make sure the material used has been wrung out sufficiently.

Cold compress - To treat
Sprains
Swellings
Headaches
Migraine
Reduce fever

Hot compress - To treat
Abscesses
Boils
Rheumatic pain (move the affected joint afterwards)
Menstrual cramp
Earache

Alternating Hot/Cold compresses - To treat
Strains
Pulled muscles

QUICK REFERENCE

1.   Room spray - Mix the essential oil in alcohol and add distilled water.

2.   Burner - night light, water and a few drops of essential oil is all that is required.

3.   Light bulb - a few drops of essential oil dropped onto a special ring which fits onto the bulb (taking care not to drop the essential oil onto the electrical fitting).

4.   Radiator - cloth soaked in water/essential oil mix and put onto a radiator.

5.   Dish - warm water. A few drops of essential oil.

6.   Cotton wool balls - Soak in cold water, wring out, add to each piece 1 drop of essential oil. Leave on open dish.

7.   Electric vapouriser

BIBLIOGRAPHY

Principles of Plant Physiology
W.E. Stiles & E.C. Cooking   Chapman Hall

Selective Toxicity - The Physico-Chemical Basis of Therapy
A. Albert   Chapman Hall

Raw Materials of Perfumery
W.A. Pouchers   Chapman Hall

Chemistry
E. Russell Harwick   Burgess
                                   Publishing Company

Horticulturists and Plant Lovers
Dr. John P Baumgardt   Timber Press

The Book of Perfumes
Eugene Rimmel

Technique of Beauty Products
R M Gattefossé & Dr H Jonquières

The Yellow Emperor's Classic of Internal Medicine
(translated by Ilza Veith in 1949)

The Herbalist
Joseph E Meyer

Aromathérapie
René-Maurice Gattefossé

Heal Thyself
Edward Bach

The Mystery & Lure of Perfume
C J S Thompson

FURTHER READING

RECOMMENDED READING OF PARTICULAR INTEREST
TO THE STUDENT OR PROFESSIONAL THERAPIST

Lecture Notes on Essential Oils
David Williams
Published by :
Eve Taylor (London) Ltd

The Essential Oil Safety Data Manual
Robert Tisserand
Published by ;
Tisserand Aromatherapy Institute

Aromatherapy An A-Z
Patricia Davis
Published by :
The C.W. Daniel Company Ltd

A Natural History of the Senses
Diane Ackerman
Published by :
Chapmans Publishers

Aromatherapy for Common Ailments
Shirley Price
Published by :
Gaia Books Ltd

USEFUL ADDRESSES

The International Society of Professional Aromatherapists (I.S.P.A.)
41 Leicester Road
Hinckley
Leicester
England
LE10 1LW

The International Federation of Aromatherapists (I.F.A.)
Department of Continuing Education
The Royal Masonic Hospital
Ravenscourt Park
London
Englan
W6 0TN

The International Examinations Board (I.E.B.)
5 Higher Drive
Banstead
Surrey
SM7 1PL
England

The International Federation of Reflexologists
78 Edridge Road
Croydon
Surrey
CR0 1EF
England

Renée Tanner is Principal of the :

Renbardou Beauty & Complementary Therapies Training Centre

Acorn House
Cherry Orchard Road
Croydon, Surrey
CR0 6BA
England

Tel : 081 686 4781

Renbardou Beauty & Complementary Therapies Training Centre

The Old School House
Multy Farnham
Co. West Meath
Ireland

Tel : 353 44 71164

Renée Tanner

Books by this author

Step By Step Anatomy & Physiology	£10.99
Step By Step Aromatherapy	£10.99
Step by Step Massage	£ 8.99
Hints & Tips on Beauty	£ 7.99
Step By Step Reflexology (2nd Edition)	£ 9.99

Video tapes (VHS) which accompany text books

Step By Step Aromatherapy	£12.99
Step By Step Introductory Massage	£12.99
Step By Step Reflexology	£12.99
Step by Step Facial Massage	£12.99
(Clense, Tone, Moisturise, Massage)	

All the above titles are available at your local bookshop or can be ordered direct from the publisher at the address below

Please send your cheque or postal order plus 75p per item to cover postage and packaging to :

Douglas Barry Publications
21 Laud Street
Croydon
Surrey
CR0 1SU
ENGLAND

Please allow twenty eight days for delivery

Acne — Bergamot — Geranium
Lavender — Sandalwood

Relaxation —

Bed wetting — Chamomile / Lavender.

Dandruff — Chamomile   Clary sage
Cedarwood — Rosemary
Lavender — TEA tree.

Cystitis Bergamot — Chamomile
Sandal wood — tea tree.
(Abdom & lower back)

Anxiety Chamomile, Clary sage
Frankensense Neroli
Sandal wood Geranium —

Arthritis (Sesame oil) Marjoram
Chamomile.
+
Rosemary + Lavender.